ARRHYTHMIAS AS EASY AS 1 2 3

The Ultimate Introductory Guide to Understanding, Diagnosing, and Treating Arrhythmias

Glenn N. Levine, MD, FACC, FAHA

Arrhythmias As Easy As 1-2-3:
The Ultimate Introductory Guide to Understanding, Diagnosing, and Treating Arrhythmias

ISBN 978-1-7348720-3-3 (paperback)
ISBN 978-1-7348720-1-9 (eBook)

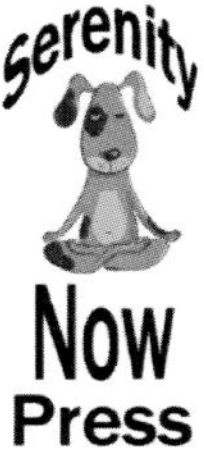

Now
Press

Glenn N. Levine, MD, FACC, FAHA
Master Clinician and Professor of Medicine,
Baylor College of Medicine

Chief, Section of Cardiology
Michael E. DeBakey VA Medical Center

Dedication

Dedicated to Lydia, who a decade ago launched me on a wonderful journey towards a better, more balanced, and more peaceful approach to life, and who continues to inspire me to try to be a better husband, friend, and person.

Contents

Introduction 1
Chapter 1 Normal Depolarization of the Heart 5
Chapter 2 Abnormal Depolarization of the Heart and Arrhythmias 9
Chapter 3 Introduction to Tachyarrhythmias 15
Chapter 4 Tachyarrhythmias Originating in the Atria 17
Chapter 5 Tachyarrhythmias That Involve the AV Node 31
Chapter 6 Tachyarrhythmias Originating in the Ventricles 41
Chapter 7 Diagnosing Tachyarrhythmias —General Approach 47
Chapter 8 Diagnosing Tachyarrhythmias —Narrow Complex Regular Tachycardia 51
Chapter 9 Diagnosing Tachyarrhythmias —Narrow Complex Irregular Tachycardia 57
Chapter 10 Diagnosing Tachyarrhythmias —Wide Complex Tachycardia 61
Chapter 11 Bradyarrhythmias and Heart Block 69
Chapter 12 Diagnosing Bradyarrhythmias 81
Chapter 13 Paced Rhythms 87
Chapter 14 Miscellaneous Arrhythmias 95
Chapter 15 BLS and ACLS Treatment of Arrhythmias 101
Chapter 16 Summary 115

Acknowledgments 119
About the Author 121

Introduction

I wrote this book with the goal of making it the most easy-to-read and understandable introductory book on understanding, recognizing, and diagnosing arrhythmias. All health-care professionals—be they physicians, nurses, nurse practitioners, physician assistants, or emergency medical personnel, will at some point have to care for the patient who develops an arrhythmia, and (hopefully!) be able to diagnose what the arrhythmia is and, in some cases, expeditiously treat it. The goal of this book is to give you enough of an understanding of arrhythmias that you can recognize what the arrhythmia is and initiate, when indicated, treatment of the patient. The sixteen chapters in this book are designed to allow you to quickly and easily achieve this goal.

As the subtitle of this book promises, diagnosing arrhythmias can be as easy as one, two, three. For example, as I discuss in greater detail, the source of all tachyarrhythmias involves one of three parts of the heart:

1. The atria
2. The AV node
3. The ventricles

Similarly, all tachyarrhythmias can be broken into one of three categories:

1. Narrow complex regular tachycardias
2. Narrow complex irregular tachycardias
3. Wide complex tachycardias

As we will discuss and review, there are six narrow complex regular tachycardias, three narrow complex irregular tachycardias, and two basic wide complex tachycardias (Figure 0.1). (There are technically a few more wide complex tachycardias that I mention in later chapters, but these are not essential for a basic understanding of arrhythmias.)

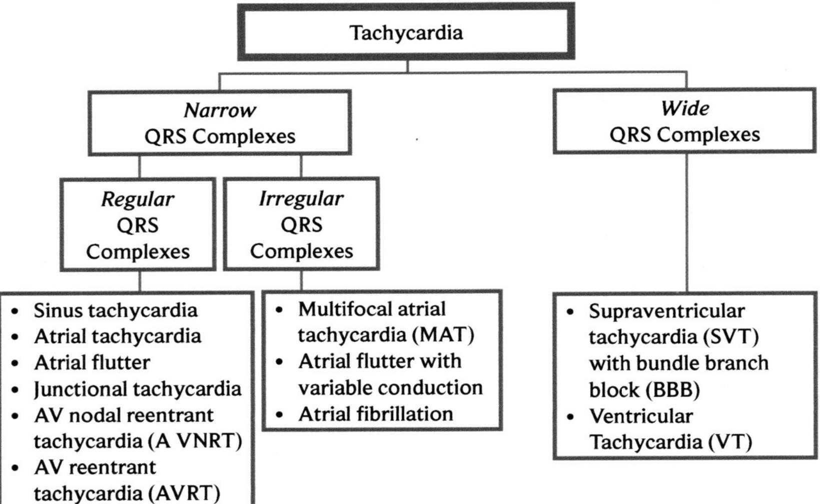

FIGURE 0.1. The three types of tachycardias: (1) narrow complex regular tachycardias, (2) narrow complex irregular tachycardias, and (3) wide complex tachycardias.

To diagnose any tachyarrhythmia, we will go over how one can use this simple three-step algorithm:

1. Determine if the QRS complexes seen in the arrhythmia are narrow or wide.
2. Determine if the QRS complexes are occurring at regular or irregular intervals
3. Determine if there is any evidence of P waves or atrial activity present.

In the coming chapters, we will discuss this three step process in more detail, and how one can use this three-step algorithm to diagnose tachyarrhythmias (Figure 0.2).

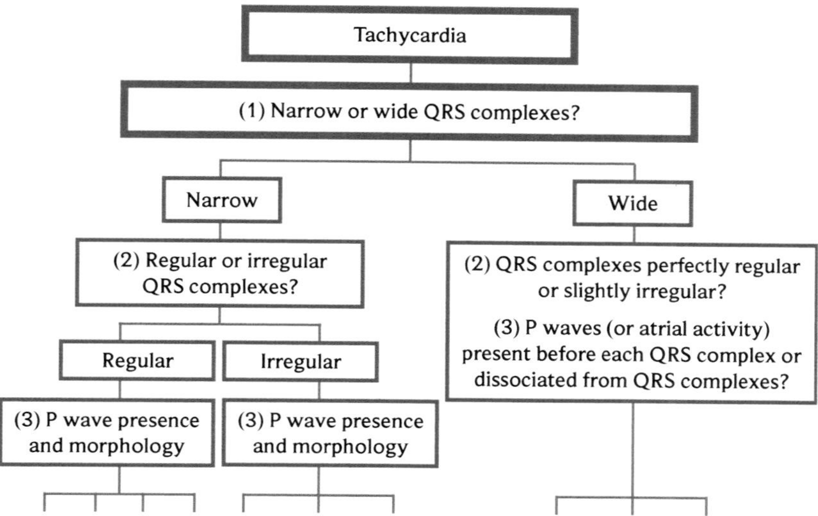

FIGURE 0.2. The three steps to diagnose any tachycardia: (1) determine if the QRS complexes seen in the arrhythmia are narrow or wide; (2) determine if the QRS complexes are occurring at regular or irregular intervals; (3) determine if there is any evidence of P waves or atrial activity present (and for wide complex tachycardias determine if the P waves dissociated from the QRS complexes).

Along the same lines, we see that heart block can be divided or categorized into one of three types:

1. First-degree heart block (slower than normal conduction of P waves into the ventricle, with a prolonged PR interval)
2. Second-degree heart block (occasional non-conducted P waves)
3. Third-degree (or complete) heart block (no conduction of P waves into the ventricle)

Just as with tachyarrhythmias, all bradyarrhythmias can be broken into one of three categories:

1. Sinus bradycardia
2. Junctional or ventricular escape rhythm due to failure of the sinoatrial (SA) node to depolarize (ie, no P waves)

3. Heart block (either second- or third-degree heart block)

And, just as we can diagnose any tachycardia, we can diagnose any bradyarrhythmias in three easy steps that I will discuss and explain:

1. Are there P waves a normal distance before each QRS complex?
   → *If so, the rhythm is sinus bradycardia.*
2. Are there no P waves a normal distance before each QRS complex?
   → *If so, the rhythm will likely be junctional rhythm.*
3. Are there more P waves than QRS complexes?
   → *If so, the rhythm is either second-degree or complete heart block.*

Don't worry about trying to memorize any of this now; we go through it in detail in later chapters.

In addition to covering the basics of arrhythmia causes, diagnosis, and treatment, I have included additional information as clinical pearls, introduced through "Heartman" (Figure 0.3).

I have used much of the information, illustrations, and methods of arrhythmia diagnoses contained in this book in the many lectures I have given over the last several decades to medical students, residents, internists, nurses, physician assistants, and other health-care professionals. I hope the book proves as useful to you as the information contained in it has been to me in teaching current and future health-care professionals. I welcome comments and suggestions from readers.

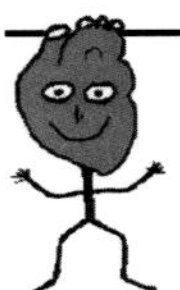

Heartman's Clinical Pearl

FIGURE 0.3. Heartman offers clinical pearls throughout the book on diagnosing and treating arrhythmias.

CHAPTER 1

Normal Depolarization of the Heart

Before we can discuss arrhythmias, we need to briefly review the parts of the heart or, more specifically, the electric and conduction system of the heart that are involved in the normal depolarization of the heart. Depolarization of the heart can be broken into three steps:

1. Depolarization of the sinoatrial (SA) node and impulse conduction down the atria
2. Depolarization impulse conduction through the atrioventricular (AV) node
3. Depolarization conduction into and throughout the ventricles via the His-Purkinje system, which includes the left bundle branch (LBB) and the right bundle branch (RBB)

Depolarization of the heart begins in the SA node, which is in the right atrium. The SA node spontaneously depolarizes, generating a depolarization impulse that travels down the heart and depolarizes the heart. The SA node normally spontaneously depolarizes 60–100 times per minute, leading to the normal heart rate of 60–100 beats per minute (commonly abbreviated as beats/min). The rhythm that results from normal depolarization of the heart is not surprisingly called "normal sinus rhythm".

After the SA node depolarizes, the depolarization impulse travels down and across the atria, depolarizing the right and left atria, and arrives at the AV node. The impulse is briefly delayed in the

AV node, contributing to the delay seen on the ECG between the P wave and the QRS complex.

Once the depolarization impulse passes through the AV node, it then makes its way into and throughout the ventricles. The depolarization impulse first passes through specialized cells called the "His Bundle" (or "Bundle of His"), which is located near the junction of the atria and ventricles. The depolarization impulse then travels down the left and right bundle branches to the ventricles. The depolarization impulse is then distributed to the cells of the left and right ventricle by specialized cells called "Purkinje fibers". The "His-Purkinje system" refers to all the specialized cells that conduct the depolarization impulse into and throughout the ventricles, and includes the His Bundle, the left and right bundle branches, and the Purkinje fibers. In simplified terms, think of the LBB as responsible for depolarization of the left ventricle and the RBB responsible for depolarization of the right ventricle (Figure 1.1).

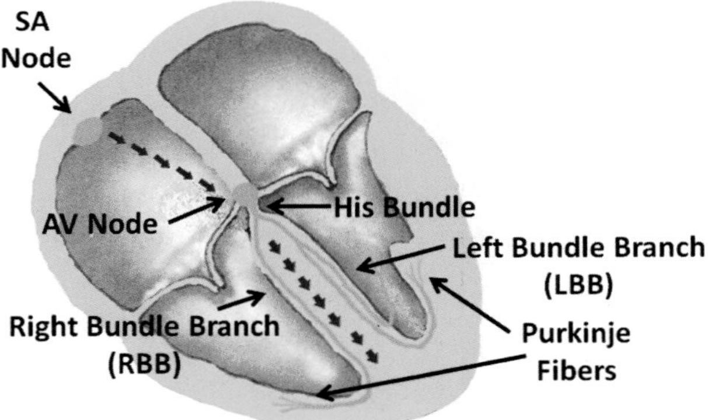

FIGURE 1.1. Normal depolarization of the heart. Spontaneous depolarization of the SA node leads to a depolarization impulse traveling down the atria to the AV node. The depolarization impulse then travels through the His Bundle and down the left bundle branch (LBB) and right bundle branch (RBB and is distributed to the cells of the ventricles via the Purkinje fibers. The His-Purkinje system denotes the system of specialized cells that transmit the depolarization impulse into and throughout the ventricles, and includes the His Bundle, the left and right bundle branches, and the Purkinje fibers.

As we will discuss in other chapters, although the SA node is the normal "pacemaker" of the heart, if spontaneous depolarization of the SA node dramatically slows or stops completely, other parts of the heart and conduction system can assume the role of the heart's pacemaker. Also, if other parts of the heart begin to abnormally and spontaneously depolarize at a rate faster than that of the SA node, then that part of the heart takes over as the heart's pacemaker.

CHAPTER 2

Abnormal Depolarization of the Heart and Arrhythmias

While the SA node is the usual pacemaker in the heart, other tissues in the heart can spontaneously depolarize, taking over as the pacemaker of the heart. Normally, the depolarization rate of the SA node is faster than the depolarization rate of other tissues. However, on occasion, other tissue in the heart will begin to spontaneously depolarize at a fast rate, faster than the rate of SA node depolarization, and take over as the pacemaker of the heart.

An abnormal and fast heart rhythm (anything >100 beats/min) is called a "tachyarrhythmia". Again, we can conceptualize tachyarrhythmias as resulting from one of three mechanisms:

1. Enhanced automaticity
2. Reentrant circuit
3. Triggered automaticity

These first two mechanisms are the most common and important for you to be aware of and understand.

When tissue in the heart begins to abnormally depolarize on its own at a fast rate, this phenomenon is referred to as "enhanced automaticity". Enhanced automaticity is the cause of some arrhythmias we will discuss, including multifocal atrial tachycardia (MAT), junctional tachycardia, most cases of atrial tachycardia, and some cases of ventricular tachycardia. Factors that can lead to enhanced automaticity include mechanical stretch of myocytes (the heart muscle cells), beta-adrenergic (eg, adrenaline, epinephrine) stimulation, and hypokalemia.

The other basic mechanism by which many tachyarrhythmias occur is that of a reentrant circuit. A reentrant circuit denotes any arrhythmia in which an electrical depolarization impulse repeatedly goes around and around part of the heart, causing an arrhythmia. Reentrant circuits can form in ischemic tissue, infarcted (dead) heart tissue, around aneurysms, and even within the AV node. A reentrant circuit can also form in patients who have Wolff-Parkinson-White (WPW) syndrome, in which there is a bypass tract (more on this in a later chapter). Reentrant circuits are the cause of some tachyarrhythmias, including AV nodal reentrant tachycardia (AVNRT), AV nodal tachycardia (AVRT), atrial flutter, many cases of ventricular tachycardia (VT), and a few cases of atrial tachycardia. (Don't try to memorize this now. We will discuss tachyarrhythmias in the next several chapters in greater detail.)

Figure 2.1 illustrates the two most common causes of tachyarrhythmias, enhanced automaticity and reentrant circuits. Atrial tachycardia is one of the few rhythms that can be causes by both enhanced automaticity and by a reentrant circuit.

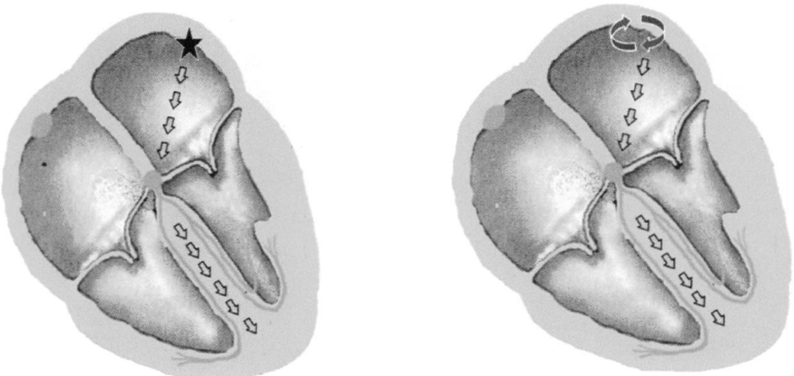

FIGURE 2.1. The two most common causes of tachyarrhythmias: enhanced automaticity (left) and reentrant circuit (right).

Heartman's Clinical Pearl

A third mechanism that can cause some arrhythmias is called "triggered automaticity". Triggered automaticity occurs when a second depolarization impulse occurs prematurely. Triggered automaticity can occur in the setting of excessive adrenergic activity, digitalis toxicity, or high intracellular calcium levels. Triggered automaticity is a rare cause of arrhythmias and is not covered in detail in this book.

Bradycardia is defined as any heart rate of <60 beats/min. Bradyarrhythmias (abnormal slow heart rates) may occur if the SA node either depolarizes at an abnormal and very slow rate or stops spontaneously depolarizing completely. In some cases, another part of the heart may take over as the pacemaker of the heart. Bradyarrhythmias may also occur if heart block develops due to dysfunction of the AV node and conduction system.

Drugs that can decrease spontaneous depolarization of the SA node and that also slow or block conduction through the AV node include beta blockers, certain calcium channel blockers (verapamil and diltiazem), digoxin, and many antiarrhythmic agents (such as amiodarone).

Medications are not always to blame for dysfunction of the SA node as the heart's pacemaker. The SA node can also become diseased over time and lose the ability to spontaneously depolarize at a normal rate. Severe hypothyroidism can also lead to sinus bradycardia. We will discuss the causes of bradyarrhythmias more in Chapter 11.

There are three (again three, hence the name of this book) parts of the heart that perform as or can assume the role of the heart's pacemaker:

1. The SA node
2. The AV node or junction
3. The myocytes (heart muscle cells) in the ventricles

It is usually the SA node, depolarizing at a rate of 60–100 beats/min, which functions as the heart's pacemaker. However, if the SA node becomes diseased or is slowed by medications, two other areas of the heart may assume the duty of pacemaker of the heart. One area is the AV node. If the AV node takes over as the pacemaker of the heart, the rhythm is called a junctional rhythm, since the AV node is located near the junction of the atria and the ventricles. Depolarization of the AV node usually occurs at a rate of 40–60 beats/min. Depolarization impulses produced by the AV node travel down the His-Purkinje system, so there is normal depolarization of the ventricles, resulting in a narrow QRS complex. Thus, junctional rhythms usually occur at a rate of 40–60 beats/min and produce a narrow QRS complex.

If both the SA node and AV node fail as pacemakers of the heart, or if there is complete heart block, tissue in the ventricles may assume the role of pacemaker of the heart. The usual rate of spontaneous depolarization of this ventricular tissue is 30–40 beats/min. Since the wave of depolarization initiated by depolarization of this ventricular tissue spreads slowly across the ventricles cell to cell, instead of via the His-Purkinje system, the resulting QRS complex is wide. Thus, a ventricular rhythm usually appears as wide QRS complexes at a rate of 30–40 beats/min.

These slow rhythms that result from spontaneous depolarization of the ventricles are called "ventricular rhythms". You may also hear this referred to as a "ventricular escape rhythm", which, in essence, means that neither the SA note nor AV node are depolarizing and only the ventricular tissue is left to become the pacemaker of the heart. Importantly, spontaneous depolarization of ventricular tissue does not always occur, and if neither the SA node nor AV node is able to spontaneously depolarize, or there is high-degree heart block, the patient may develop asystole (meaning there is no contraction of the ventricles) (Figure 2.2). That is not good! We will discuss this further in Chapter 11.

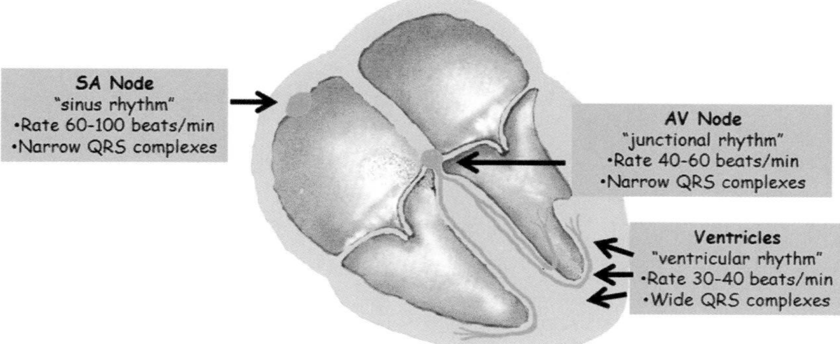

FIGURE 2.2. If the SA node fails as the pacemaker of the heart, the AV node or tissue in the ventricle may assume the role of the heart's pacemaker.

CHAPTER 3

Introduction to Tachyarrhythmias

A tachycardia is by definition any heart rhythm at a rate >100 beats/min. A tachyarrhythmia is any *abnormal* heart rhythm that leads to a heart rate greater than 100 beats/min. As we discussed in the introduction, the source of all tachyarrhythmias can be broken down as involving one of three parts of the heart:

1. The atria
2. The AV node
3. The ventricles

Tachycardias and tachyarrhythmias that occur in the atria include:

- Sinus tachycardia
- Atrial tachycardia
- Multifocal atrial tachycardia (MAT)
- Atrial flutter
- Atrial fibrillation

Tachyarrhythmias that involve the AV node include:

- Junctional tachycardia
- AV nodal reentrant tachycardia (AVNRT)
- AV reentrant tachycardia (AVNT)

Tachyarrhythmias that originate in the ventricles include:

- Ventricular tachycardia (VT)
- Torsade de Pointes (a special type of ventricular tachycardia)

- Ventricular fibrillation (VF)

Figure 3.1 demonstrates this useful way of conceptualizing the cause of tachyarrhythmias based upon where in the heart they originate from or what part of the heart they involve. This will hopefully make it easier to understand and remember the different tachycardias, rather than just memorizing a long list of different arrhythmias.

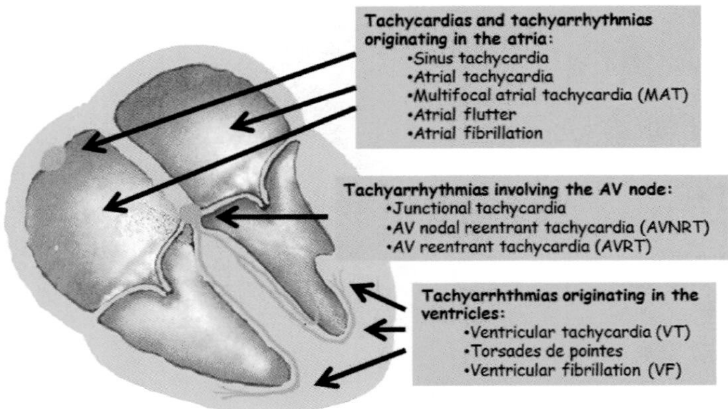

FIGURE 3.1. Parts of the heart involved in tachyarrhythmias.

In the simplest terms, tachycardias are classified as either "supraventricular tachycardias" or "ventricular tachycardias". Any tachycardia that is caused by a rhythm abnormality originating in the atria or involving the AV node is called a supraventricular (above the ventricle) tachycardia (SVT). Tachycardias that develop in the ventricle are ventricular tachycardias (VT).

In the following three chapters we will review the different heart rhythms that cause tachycardias and tachyarrhythmias, starting at the "top" of the heart in the atria and working down to the ventricles.

CHAPTER 4

Tachyarrhythmias Originating in the Atria

In this chapter we will discuss the tachycardias that originate in the atria of the heart. Not surprisingly, these arrhythmias are called "atrial arrhythmias". These rhythms include:

- Sinus tachycardia
- Atrial tachycardia
- Multifocal atrial tachycardia (MAT)
- Atrial flutter
- Atrial fibrillation

Sinus Tachycardia

Although sinus tachycardia is not technically an arrhythmia, it is important to briefly discuss sinus tachycardia, as it can be mistaken for a pathological arrhythmia, and because when it occurs, it is important to figure out what is *causing* the sinus tachycardia. The ECG in Figure 4.1 shows an example of sinus tachycardia. If you don't recognize that there are P waves before each QRS complex, this rhythm could be mistaken for a pathological tachyarrhythmia.

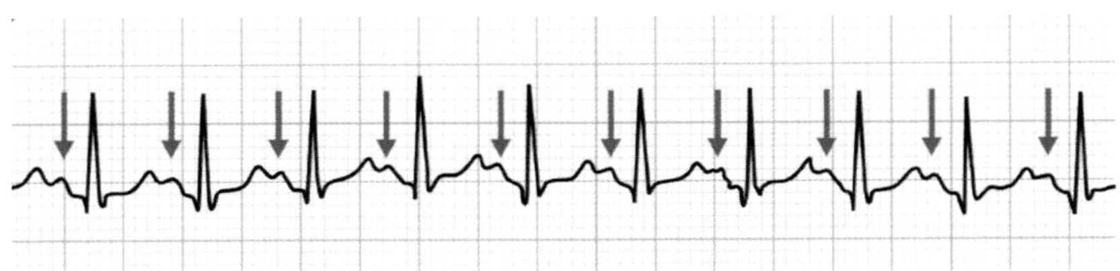

FIGURE 4.1. Sinus tachycardia. If you do not see there are P waves before each QRS complex, this rhythm could be mistaken for an arrhythmia.

Sinus tachycardia is, in general, caused by increased sympathetic stimulation of the SA node in response to some stressor on the body. Stressors that can cause a sinus tachycardia are listed in Table 4.1. It is important to be able to remember all these possible causes when trying to come up with a differential diagnosis of why a person has a new or persistent sinus tachycardia.

TABLE 4.1. Stressors that can cause a sinus tachycardia.

• Fever
• Anxiety or pain
• Hypoxemia
• Severe anemia
• Hypotension from acute bleeding, dehydration, or sepsis
• Heart failure or overt cardiogenic shock
• Pericardial tamponade
• Tension pneumothorax
• Pulmonary embolism
• Medications or medication overdose
• Hyperthyroidism

Heartman's Clinical Pearl

Remember, since sinus tachycardia is almost always a physiological response to some stress, you almost never try to simply treat the tachycardia itself (such as with medications that slow SA node depolarization like a beta blocker). Rather, the key is to identify and treat the ***underlying*** *cause of the sinus tachycardia in patients with a new or persistent sinus tachycardia.*

Atrial Tachycardia

Atrial tachycardia is an arrhythmia that originates in the right or left atrium at a site other than where the SA node is located. Most commonly, atrial tachycardia is due to a focal area of tissue that begins to spontaneously depolarize at an abnormal fast rate (as shown in the left of Figure 4.2). When a part of the heart begins to spontaneously depolarize at an abnormally fast rate, it is called "enhanced automaticity". Atrial tachycardia may also occasionally occur when a reentrant circuit develops in the atria (as shown in the right of Figure 4.2). A "reentrant circuit" denotes any arrhythmia in which an electrical impulse repeatedly goes around and around part of the heart, causing an arrhythmia.

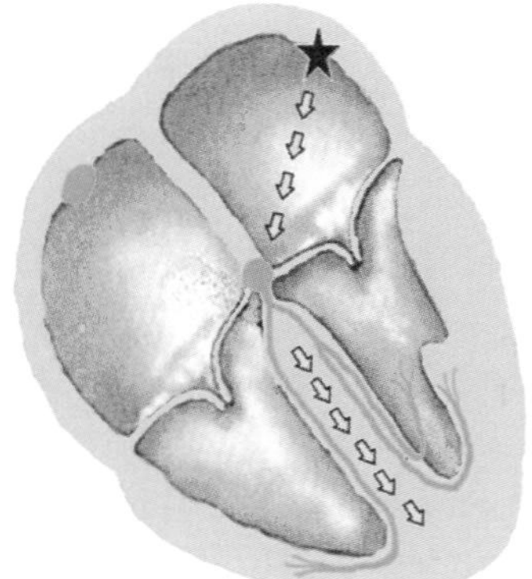

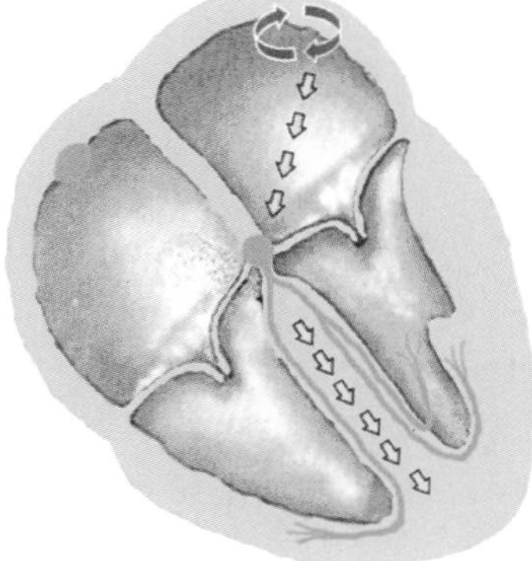

FIGURE 4.2. Atrial tachycardia is usually caused by enhanced automaticity of an area of atrial tissue (left) but on occasion can be due to a reentrant circuit forming in the atria (right).

Whether the arrhythmia is caused by enhanced automaticity or a reentrant circuit, the depolarization impulse spreads across the atria, leading to depolarization of the atria. Depolarization of the atria leads to a P wave being seen on the ECG. However, because the atria are depolarized in a pattern different from that during sinus rhythm, the P waves appear different in morphology from those seen during sinus rhythm. Depending upon where in the atria the arrhythmia originates, the P waves in some leads may appear inverted (as shown by the arrows in the rhythm strip in Figure 4.3). The depolarization impulse continues down the AV node and into the ventricles. Depolarization of the ventricles leads to QRS complexes being seen on the ECG. Thus, in atrial tachycardia, we see abnormal or inverted P waves before each QRS complex (Figure 4.3).

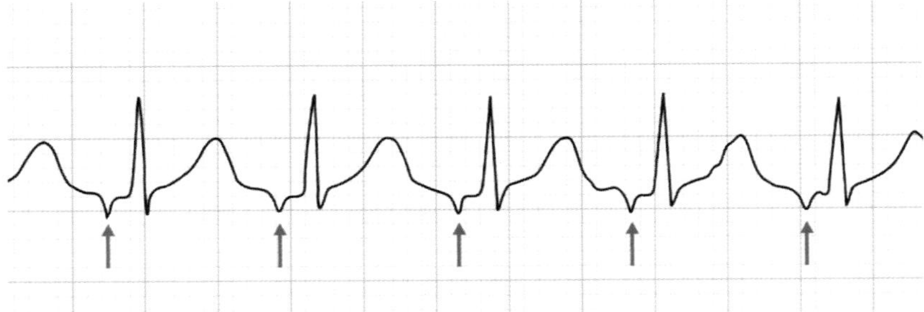

FIGURE 4.3. The ECG seen with atrial tachycardia. The P wave morphology with atrial tachycardia is different from the P waves that are seen with normal sinus rhythm. Here, they appear "inverted."

Although the rate of atrial tachycardia can vary anywhere between 100–250 beats/min, the heart rate most commonly seen in patients with atrial tachycardia is in the range of 160–180 beats/min. Atrial tachycardia can occur in diseased atria or in structurally normal hearts. Atrial tachycardia may be caused by digoxin toxicity (though this is seen infrequently these days). Very short runs (<10–20 beats) of atrial tachycardia are not infrequently seen incidentally on ambulatory event monitoring and are often not associated with symptoms (other than perhaps occasional palpitations). More sustained episodes may cause symptoms in addition to palpitations, such as transient lightheadedness.

Atrial tachycardia usually resolves on its own. Antiarrhythmic agents or other medications are usually not used to try to terminate the arrhythmia or slow the ventricular response rate, since such drugs rarely acutely terminate the arrhythmia or successfully decrease impulse conduction through the AV node. Though not usually the case, atrial tachycardia is occasionally terminated by administration of adenosine. Since atrial tachycardia is more commonly the result of enhanced automaticity than of a reentrant circuit, cardioverting ("shocking") the patient usually does not terminate the arrhythmia.

Multifocal Atrial Tachycardia

Multifocal atrial tachycardia (MAT) is an arrhythmia that is caused by multiple sites of tissue in the atria depolarizing, each at a different rate and time. Each time one of these sites spontaneously depolarizes, the atria are depolarized. Because these different areas of depolarizing tissue are spontaneously depolarizing at different times, impulses reach the AV node and are conducted to the ventricles at varying intervals, leading to an irregular ventricular response rate and heartbeat (Figure 4.4).

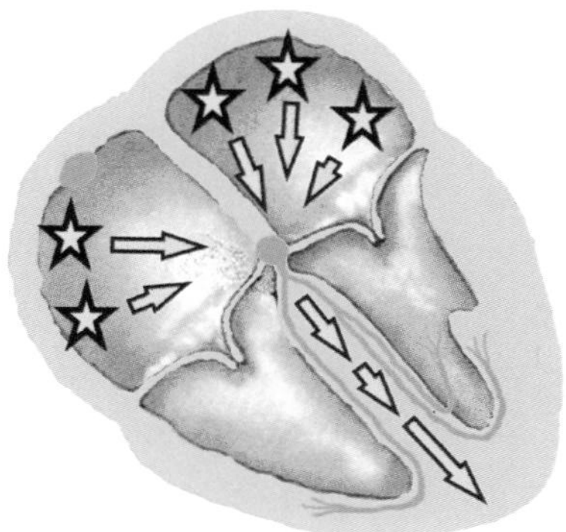

FIGURE 4.4. Multifocal atrial tachycardia (MAT). There are multiple areas in the atria in which the tissue has begun to spontaneously depolarize.

Because in MAT depolarization of the atria begins at different parts of the atria, the differing patterns of atrial depolarization lead to P waves of different morphologies (as shown by the arrows in Figure 4.5). Since spontaneous depolarization of different parts of the atria occurs at different times, the resulting rhythm is irregular (there are varying intervals between the QRS complexes). By definition, MAT is diagnosed when there are at least three distinct P wave morphologies and the heart rate is greater than 100 beats/min.

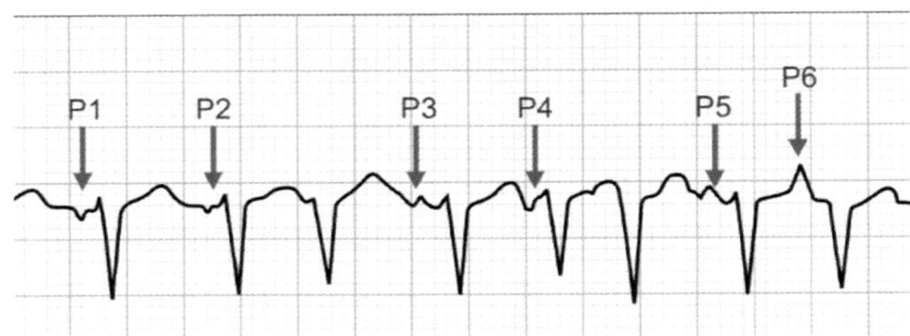

FIGURE 4.5. The ECG seen with multifocal atrial tachycardia (MAT). The rhythm is irregular and there are numerous P waves of differing morphology before each QRS complex. P1–P6 denote different P wave morphologies.

MAT most often occurs in patients with lung disease, particularly those with chronic obstructive pulmonary disease (COPD). The usual treatment for MAT is to treat the *underlying cause* that has triggered it, such as a COPD exacerbation. As with atrial tachycardia, in MAT antiarrhythmic agents or other medications are usually not used to try to terminate the arrhythmia or slow the heart rate. Since the arrhythmia is caused by enhanced automaticity of tissues in the atria and not a reentrant circuit, shocking the patient will not terminate the arrhythmia.

Atrial Flutter

Atrial flutter is another arrhythmia that occurs in the atria. An impulse travels around and around the atria in a repetitive loop, forming a reentrant loop or, more technically, a reentrant circuit. This reentrant circuit is illustrated in Figures 4.6 and 4.7.

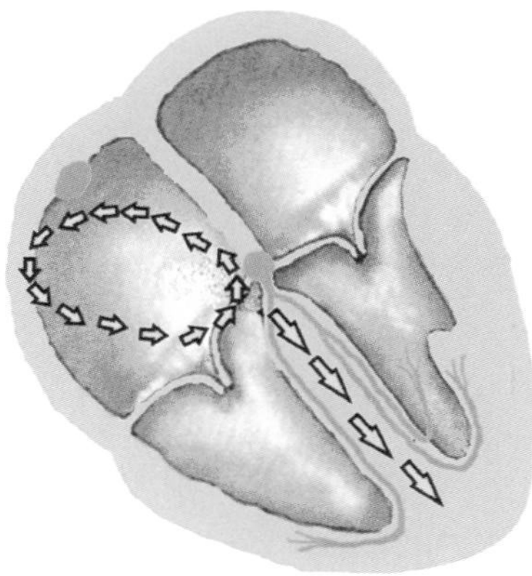

FIGURE 4.6. Atrial flutter. A reentrant circuit forms in the atria, leading to the arrhythmia.

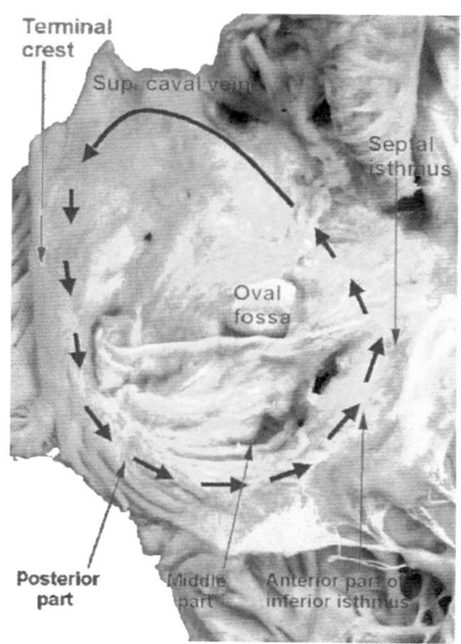

FIGURE 4.7. The actual pathway (blue arrows) that a typical atrial flutter takes as it courses around the right atrium. Image courtesy of Dr. Robert Anderson.

In most persons, the impulses travel around the reentrant circuit about 300 times per minute (though this can range from 220–350 impulses per minute). Each time the impulse travels around the reentrant circuit, it depolarizes the atria, leading to the sawtooth pattern flutter waves seen in atrial flutter (Figures 4.8 and 4.9).

FIGURE 4.8. Schematic of the sawtooth pattern caused by atrial flutter on an ECG.

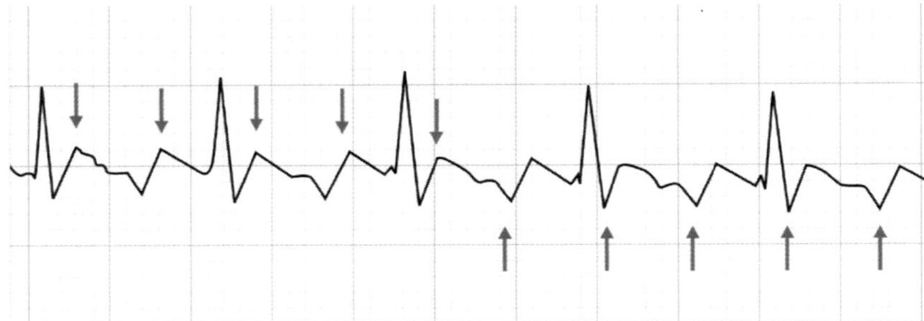

FIGURE 4.9. Actual ECG tracing of the sawtooth pattern of flutter waves that are seen in atrial flutter.

The AV node cannot conduct each of these 300 impulses per minute to the ventricle. Instead, in many persons, it conducts every other impulse down in the ventricle. When this occurs, we say that there is 2:1 AV conduction, meaning that for every two depolarizations in the atria, there is one depolarization of the ventricle. Thus, in many people who experience atrial flutter, the actual flutter rate is 300 beats/min, but the ventricular rate is 150 beats/min. In some people, if the AV node is "sick" or diseased, or if that person is on medications that slow conduction in the AV node, the AV node conducts even fewer impulses from the atria down to the ventricle. Such persons may have 3:1 conduction or even 4:1 conduction, leading to ventricular rates of 100 or 75 beats/min. In other persons, there may be a varying degree of conduction that leads to an irregular ventricular rate. (I discuss that more in a later chapter.)

Atrial flutter can occur in different parts of the atria. It most commonly occurs in a specific pathway within the right atrium. A wide spectrum of diseases is associated with the occurrence of atrial flutter. Depending on the ventricular response rate, patients may be asymptomatic or may experience symptoms such as palpitations, lightheadedness, shortness of breath, or chest discomfort.

When atrial flutter occurs, there is not the normal, forceful, contraction of the atria. Because of this, patients with atrial flutter are at risk for forming a clot (more technically a thrombus) in a part of the left atrium called the left atrial appendage. There is a small chance that such a clot can embolize into the circulation and to the brain, so patients with atrial flutter are at risk of having a stroke and are often treated with anticoagulation therapy.

There are two basic approaches to the patient with atrial flutter. If the ventricular rate is too fast, then the patient can be treated with medications that decrease conduction of impulses from the atria through the AV node into the ventricles. Medications that decrease conduction of impulses through the AV node include beta blockers (such as metoprolol, atenolol, and carvedilol), certain calcium channel blockers (diltiazem and verapamil), and digoxin. The other approach is to shock (or, more technically, electrically cardiovert) the patient out of atrial flutter and back to normal sinus rhythm.

Long-term treatment to prevent the recurrence of atrial flutter includes either the use of antiarrhythmic agents (such as amiodarone) or electrical ablation of part of the tissue involved in the reentrant circuit.

Heartman's Clinical Pearl

Atrial flutter most commonly occurs as a counterclockwise electric circuit in the right atrium (Figure 4.6). This is called "typical atrial flutter". A reentrant circuit, however, can also develop in other parts of the atria, including the left atria. Any atrial reentrant circuit other than this typical flutter circuit is called "atypical atrial flutter". In atypical atrial flutter, we may see not the typical sawtooth ECG pattern, but rather somewhat more discrete P or flutter waves. While typical atrial flutter is usually easy to ablate with high (>90—95%) acute and long-term success rates, atypical atrial flutter is often more challenging, and patients are at some longer-term risk of developing another atypical atrial flutter.

Atrial Fibrillation

Atrial fibrillation is a strange arrhythmia that also occurs in the atria. In atrial fibrillation, multiple "wavelets" of depolarization are constantly forming and reforming in the atria. As a result, there is no organized depolarization of the atria; rather than contract in any organized manner, the atria just "fibrillate." Some of the many impulses generated by these wavelets of depolarization reach the AV node, and some of these are conducted down into the ventricles. Because these depolarization impulses reach the AV node at irregular intervals, and because the AV node conducts some of these impulses to the ventricle at irregular intervals, ventricular depolarization and contraction occurs at irregular intervals. Thus, with atrial fibrillation, there is what is called an irregular ventricular response rate, similar to what we see with MAT (Figure 4.10). In some patients with a healthy AV node, the ventricular response rate can be in the range of 150–180 beats/min. In those with sicker AV nodes or those on medications that decrease conduction through the AV node, the ventricular response rate will be slower.

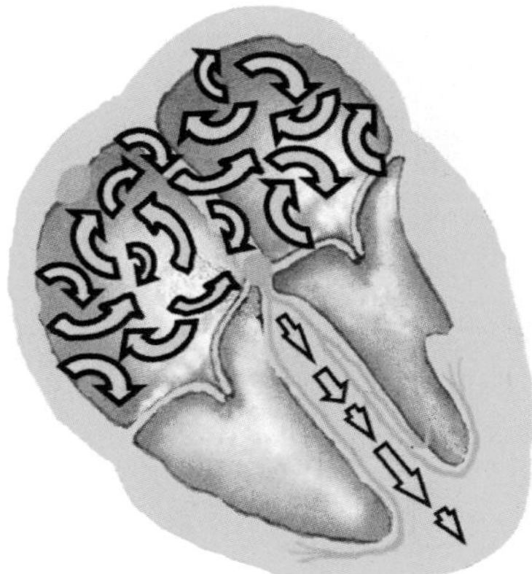

FIGURE 4.10. The multiple wavelets of depolarization impulses in atrial fibrillation.

Because in atrial fibrillation there is no organized depolarization of the atria, there are no P waves seen on the ECG (Figures 4.11 and 4.12). Rather, there are only numerous, random, and varying, small bumps (or deflections) of the ECG tracing. These varying deflections are what are called "fibrillatory waves".

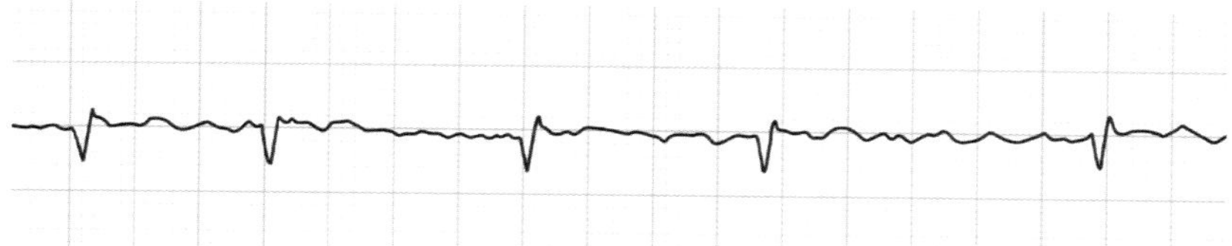

FIGURE 4.11. The ECG in atrial fibrillation. No P waves or organized atrial activity is evident. The small random deflections of the ECG baseline are due to fibrillatory waves.

There are numerous causes of atrial fibrillation. Atrial fibrillation not infrequently occurs in persons with dilated atria and in those with heart failure. Table 4.2 lists some of the important causes of atrial fibrillation to consider when you encounter a patient who has developed atrial fibrillation.

TABLE 4.2. Conditions associated with the development of atrial fibrillation.

Condition
• Dilated atria
• Heart failure and cardiomyopathy
• Acute myocardial ischemia
• Coronary artery disease
• Hypertension
• Pericarditis
• Pulmonary embolism
• Hyperthyroidism
• Toxins (including alcohol)

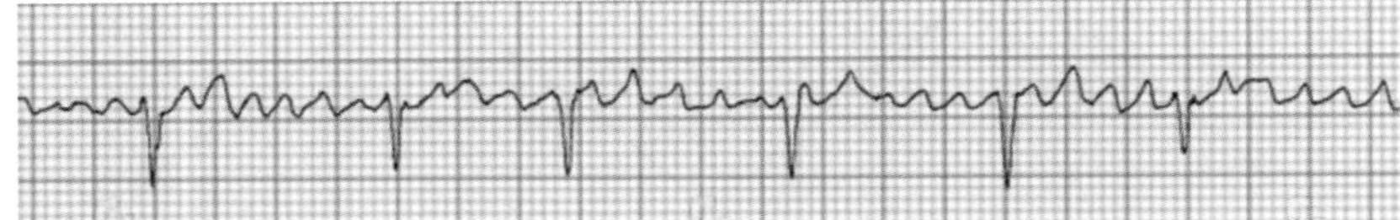

FIGURE 4.12. Another example of atrial fibrillation. Note that this might be mistaken for the flutter waves of atrial flutter. However, in atrial flutter, all the flutter waves look exactly the same. Here, there are more random deflections of various shapes and at differing rates. This is the result of random, disorganized depolarization of the atrium that we see in atrial fibrillation.

In many patients, atrial fibrillation is believed to be triggered or initiated by impulse formation in one of the four pulmonary veins that drain blood from the lungs to the left atrium. The impulse begins in the pulmonary vein and is then propagated throughout the atria, leading to atrial fibrillation. This impulse initiation and spread are illustrated in the Figure 4.13. In such patients, a procedure called a "pulmonary vein ablation" (or, more technically correct, a "pulmonary vein isolation" [PVI]) may be performed to decrease the chances of the atrial fibrillation recurring.

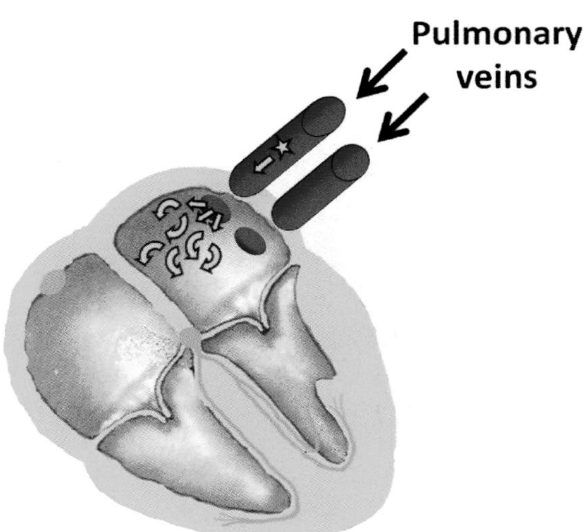

FIGURE 4.13. An impulse originating in the pulmonary vein, which then spreads to through the atria, is the cause of many cases of paroxysmal atrial fibrillation.

Since there is no organized contraction of the atria, patients with atrial fibrillation are at risk of forming a blood clot in the part of the atria called the "left atrial appendage" (Figure 4.14). As with atrial flutter, such patients have a small but real risk of having such a blood clot embolize to the brain, causing a stroke. To decrease the risk of blood clots forming in the left atrial appendage of the heart, patients with atrial fibrillation are often treated with anticoagulants such as warfarin (Coumadin) or more commonly these days the newer blood thinners called direct oral anticoagulants (DOACs) such as apixaban (Eliquis), dabigatran (Pradaxa), edoxaban (Savaysa), or rivaroxaban (Xarelto).

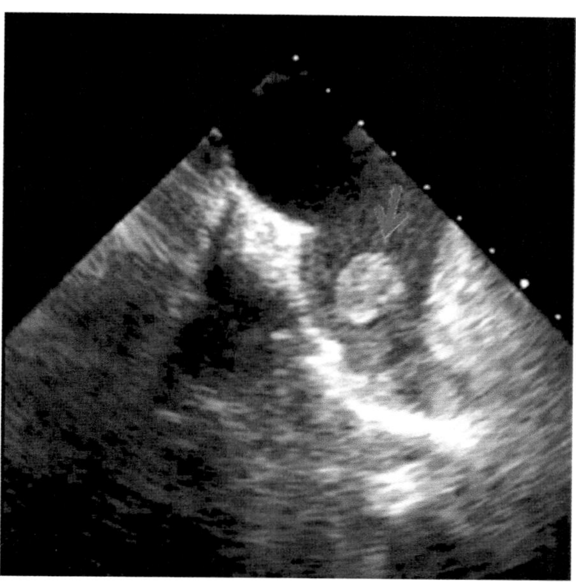

FIGURE 4.14. An image obtained during transesophageal echocardiography (TEE) showing a thrombus (clot) in the left atrial appendage (red arrow). This is why patients with atrial fibrillation and atrial flutter are put on anticoagulants to prevent such thrombus formation (and, more importantly, to prevent a thrombus from forming that can embolize to the brain, resulting in stroke).

As with atrial flutter, there are two basic approaches to the patient with atrial fibrillation. If the ventricular response rate is too fast, the patient is treated with medications that decrease conduction through the AV node, such as beta blockers, certain calcium channel blockers, and digoxin. The other approach to patients with atrial fibrillation is to shock (or more technically electrically cardiovert) the patient out of atrial fibrillation and back to normal sinus rhythm. Unfortunately, many patients who develop atrial fibrillation eventually go back into atrial fibrillation, even if successfully shocked back to normal sinus rhythm.

Antiarrhythmic drugs such as amiodarone can be used to decrease the chances that atrial fibrillation will recur, but even amiodarone long term keeps only approximately half of treated patients in sinus rhythm long term. Pulmonary vein isolation significantly decreases the chances that atrial fibrillation will recur, but it may still recur in 20%–40% of cases after the PVI procedure.

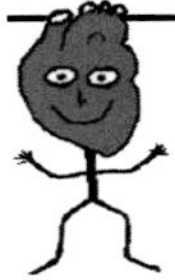

Heartman's Clinical Pearl

For those interested, atrial fibrillation (AF) can be categorized into three categories based on the following nomenclature:

1. ***Paroxysmal, episodic AF:*** *Atrial fibrillation converts spontaneously to normal sinus rhythm.*
2. ***Persistent AF:*** *Atrial fibrillation terminates only after intervention (electrical or chemical cardioversion).*
3. ***Permanent AF:*** *Atrial fibrillation resists attempts to restore normal sinus rhythm and the patient remains in AF.*

CHAPTER 5

Tachyarrhythmias That Involve the AV Node

In this chapter we will focus on the three tachyarrhythmias that involve the AV node or tissue in the area of the AV node. The three rhythms we will discuss are:

1. Junctional tachycardia
2. AV nodal reentrant tachycardia (AVNRT)
3. AV reentrant tachycardia (AVNT)

Junctional Tachycardia

As we discussed earlier in the book, tissue in the area of the AV node has the potential to spontaneously depolarize. If the SA node fails to spontaneously depolarize, this tissue may take over as the pacemaker of the heart. This rhythm, usually occurring at a rate of 40–60 beats per minute, is termed "junctional rhythm". It is also possible for this tissue to begin to spontaneously depolarize at a faster rate. If this occurs, and the resulting heart rate is 60–100 beats/min, the rhythm is termed "accelerated junctional rhythm". This tissue may occasionally begin to depolarize at a rate of >100 beats/min. When this occurs, this spontaneously depolarizing tissue usually takes over the pacemaker function of the heart. The resulting rhythm is termed "junctional tachycardia". When junctional tachycardia occurs, the resulting ECG demonstrates narrow QRS complexes at a rate of >100 beats/min; P waves are often not present

Unfortunately, different books, review articles, and websites use different terminology when discussing junctional tachycardia. Some sources use junctional tachycardia to encompass *any* rhythm that involves the AV node, including the reentrant rhythms discussed below, specifically AV nodal reentrant tachycardia (AVNRT) and AV reentrant tachycardia (AVRT). Also, while some refer to an arrhythmia due to spontaneous depolarization of the tissue around the AV node as simply junctional tachycardia, others refer to this as "ectopic junctional tachycardia", "non-paroxysmal junctional tachycardia", or "non-reentrant junctional tachycardia". This is too confusing! Thus, for our purposes, in this book we will simply use the term "junctional tachycardia" to refer to a tachyarrhythmia due to abnormal spontaneous depolarization of tissue in or around the AV node, and separately refer to other arrhythmias that may involve the AV node but involve a reentrant circuit, such as AVNRT or AVRT (Figure 5.1 and 5.2).

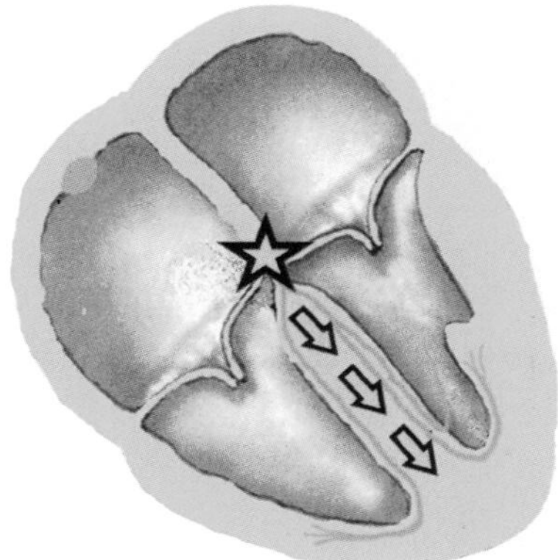

FIGURE 5.1. Junctional tachycardia. An area of tissue in or near the AV node begins to spontaneously depolarize at a rate >100 beats/min. Impulses travel from the area of spontaneous depolarization down the His-Purkinje system and into the ventricle.

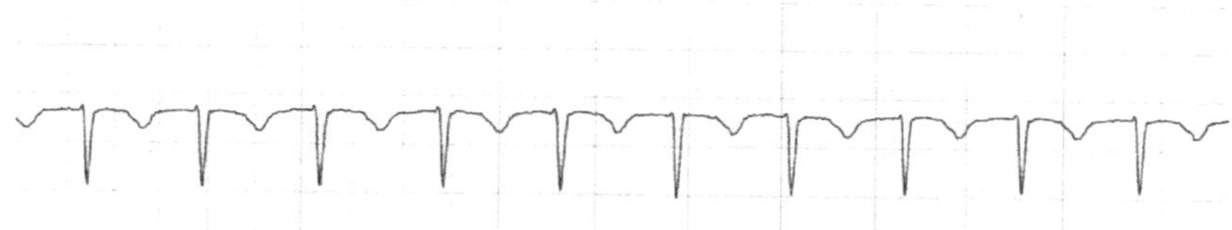

FIGURE 5.2. Junctional tachycardia. Regular narrow QRS complexes are present at a rate of 120 beats/min. No P waves are present.

Junctional tachycardia can occur in cases of digoxin toxicity, acute MI, electrolyte abnormalities (such as hypokalemia), after open heart surgery, or due to various other causes. Most commonly, the heart rate is 101–120 beats/min. Much faster (>140 beats/min) narrow complex tachycardias in which there are no P waves or flutter waves present are usually due to either AVNRT or AVRT (discussed next).

Junctional tachycardia usually does not cause the patient significant symptoms. No specific treatment is usually taken in patients who develop junctional tachycardia other than to try to determine the underlying cause of the arrhythmia.

Heartman's Clinical Pearl

We name rhythms caused by spontaneous depolarization of the tissue in or around the AV node (located at the junction of the heart between the atria and ventricles) based upon the heart rate, breaking these down into three named rhythms:

1. *Heart rate 40–60 beats/min = junctional rhythm*
2. *Heart rate 61–100 beats/min = accelerated junctional rhythm*
3. *Heart rate >100 beats/min = junctional tachycardia*

AV Nodal Reentrant Tachycardia

AV nodal reentrant tachycardia (AVNRT) is an arrhythmia that takes place in the area of the AV node, as shown in Figure 5.3. Within the AV node, two impulse-conducting pathways exist. In AVNRT, the impulse goes down one pathway and then up the other in a repetitive loop or circuit. Each time the impulse circles around, an impulse leading to depolarization is sent down the His-Purkinje system into the ventricles, leading to ventricular depolarization.

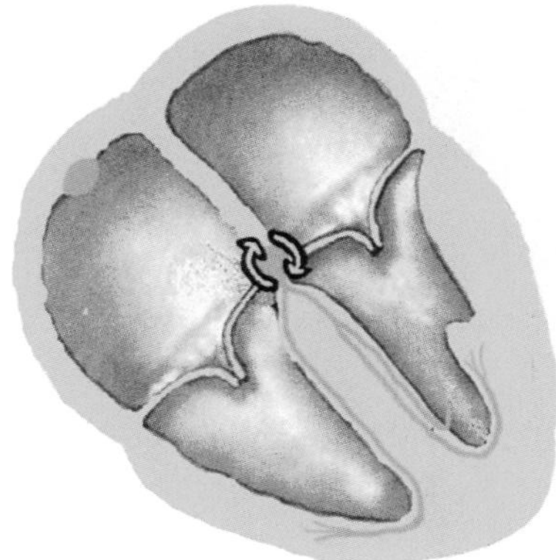

FIGURE 5.3. AV Nodal Reentrant Tachycardia (AVNRT). A reentrant circuit forms in the area of the AV node.

Each time the impulse circles around the AV node, a depolarizing impulse may also proceed up into the atria, leading to atrial depolarization as well. Atrial depolarization occurs at the same time or just after ventricular depolarization. Because of this, the P waves caused by atrial depolarization are often "buried" or "hidden" in the QRS complex and not seen on an ECG tracing, or P waves are seen occurring at the end of or just after the QRS complex. Because atrial depolarization occurs from the bottom of the atria to the top of the atria, instead of the normal top-to-bottom depolarization, the P waves appear inverted in some leads of the ECG (arrows in Figure 5.4).

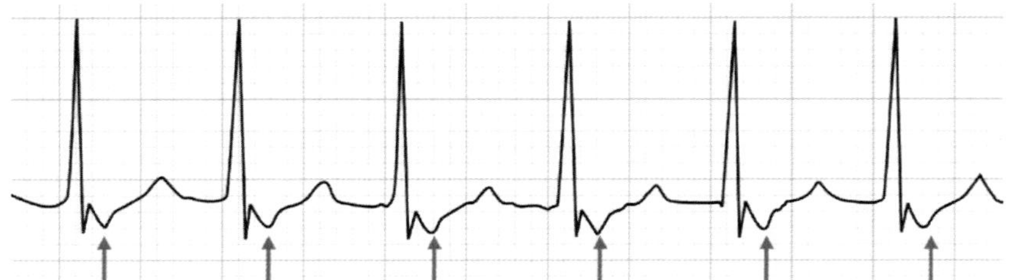

FIGURE 5.4. An example of AVNRT with small retrograde, inverted P waves (arrows) occurring immediately after the QRS complexes.

Although AVNRT occurs at a rate of anywhere from 120–250 beats/min, most patients who develop AVNRT have a heart rate of about 160–200 beats/min. The most common symptom that patients experience is palpitations. AVNRT can develop in patients without any heart disease, and occasionally is a cause of palpitations in otherwise healthy persons.

AVNRT is not due to structural heart disease (such as dilated atrial or ventricles) or to ischemic heart disease (coronary artery disease or old MI). Rather, it is simply an electrical disease of the heart. These rhythms are often initiated by a premature atrial contraction (PAC) or a premature ventricular contraction (PVC).

Initial treatment involves administering medications that slow conduction in the AV node, which can terminate the reentrant arrhythmia and prevent its recurrence. Adenosine is a short-acting intravenous drug that is frequently used to terminate AVNRT. Beta blockers and certain calcium channel blockers are used to both break the arrhythmia and to prevent its occurrence. In some patients in whom AVNRT repeatedly recurs, a procedure called "catheter ablation" will be performed.

AV Reentrant Tachycardia

In one to three out of every 1,000 persons, in addition to the normal conduction system, the heart has an accessory bypass tract. This accessory bypass tract quickly conducts impulses from the atria to the ventricles, bypassing the AV node and His-Purkinje system. The bypass tract also conducts impulses in the other direction, from the ventricles into the atria. Patients who have a bypass tract like this are said to have Wolff-Parkinson-White (WPW) syndrome.

In AV reentrant tachycardia (AVRT), a reentrant circuit can be formed when an impulse goes through the AV node and down the His-Purkinje system in to the ventricle, then up the bypass tract into the atria, and then again back down the AV node and His-Purkinje system, forming a repetitive loop or circuit (Figure 5.5). When the impulse in the reentrant circuit travels in this manner, the QRS complexes appear narrow since ventricular depolarization is occurring via the His-Purkinje system in an organized manner. This pattern of impulse conduction is called "orthodromic conduction", though don't worry about memorizing this fancy term unless you really want to.

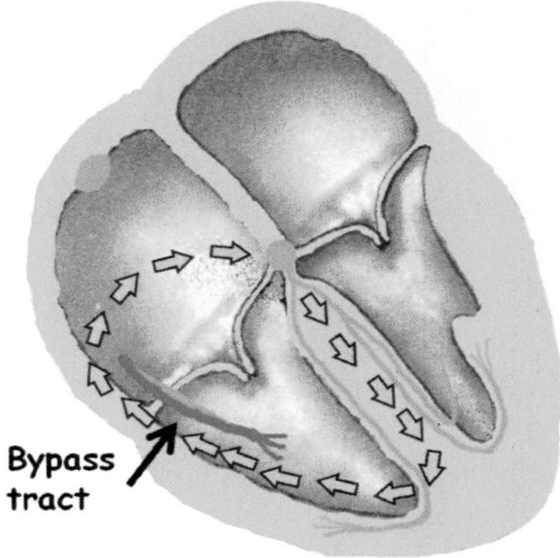

FIGURE 5.5. In AVRT a bypass tract becomes part of a reentrant loop. This pattern of impulse conduction is called "orthodromic conduction and results in narrow QRS complexes occurring at a regular rate.

In AVRT, atrial depolarization occurs after ventricular depolarization. Thus, in some cases, P waves can be seen occurring after the QRS complex, often in the ST segment or T wave (Figure 5.6). As in the case with AVNRT, because atrial depolarization is occurring in a bottom-to-top direction, the P waves appear inverted in some leads (Figure 5.7). In not all cases of AVRT, though, will such P waves be visible. On some ECG tracings, all we see are QRS complexes.

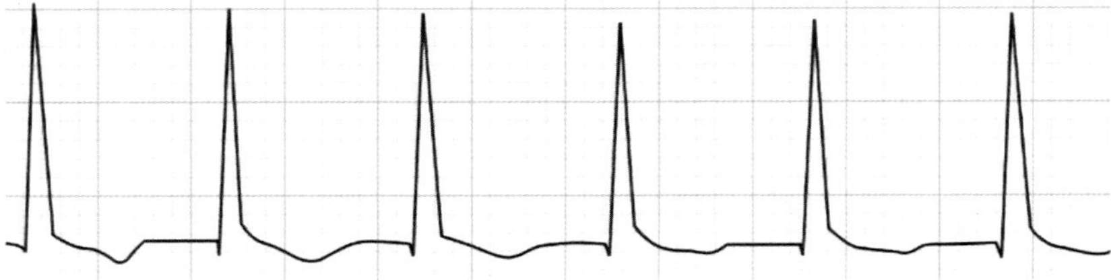

FIGURE 5.6. An example of the ECG that can be seen in AVRT. No P waves are present before the QRS complexes, as would occur with sinus rhythm. While in AVRT P waves can sometimes be seen occurring after the QRS complex, none are visible on this ECG.

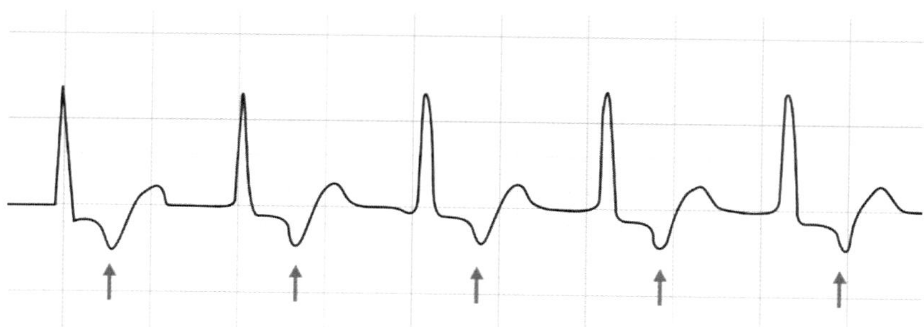

FIGURE 5.7. An example of AVRT in which retrograde P waves occurring after the QRS complexes are visible. Notice how the inverted P waves distort the ST segments.

The presence of a bypass tract can be recognized by three findings on the 12-lead ECG:

1. Short PR interval
2. Wide QRS complex
3. Initial slow upstroke of the QRS complex called a "delta wave"

These findings are shown in Figure 5.8, and were classically described by the persons for whom this syndrome is named, Wolff, Parkinson, and White (Figure 5.9).

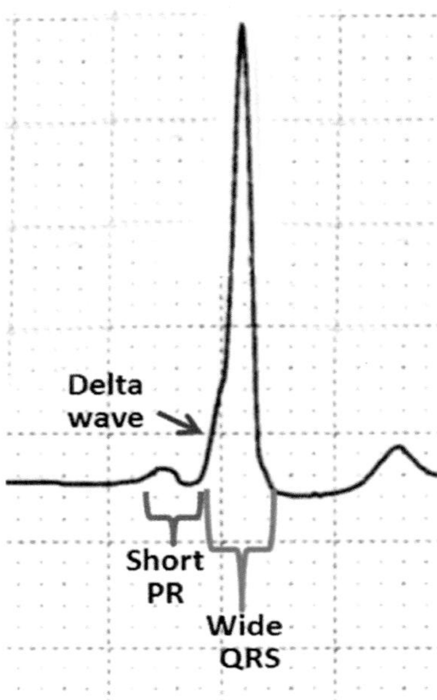

FIGURE 5.8. The three findings on ECG that suggest the presence of an accessory bypass tract, such as described in WPW: (1) short PR interval; (2) wide QRS complex; and (3) initial slow upstroke of the QRS complex, a delta wave.

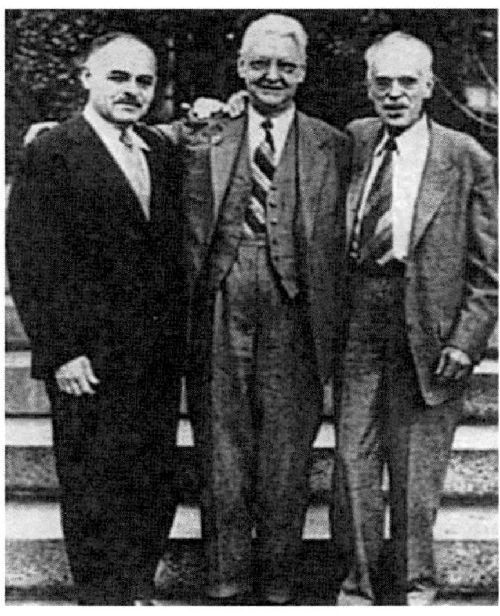

FIGURE 5.9. Louis Wolff, John Parkinson, and Paul Dudley White who described the ECG findings in 1930. Image from Wikipedia.

Rarely, a reentrant circuit can also be formed in which the depolarization impulse travels from the atria through the bypass track into the ventricle and then up the His-Purkinje system, through the AV node, and back up to the atria (the reverse direction as shown in Figure 5.8). The technical term for this type of conduction pattern is "antidromic conduction" (don't bother memorizing this fancy term). This is a rarer form of AVRT reentrant circuit, occurring only in 5%–10% of cases of AVRT (Figure 5.10). In this case, because the His-Purkinje system is not involved in depolarizing the ventricles, ventricular depolarization takes longer as the depolarization impulse must travel across the ventricle myocyte to myocyte, and the QRS complexes appear wide. This rare arrhythmia can thus be mistaken for ventricular tachycardia (Figure 5.11).

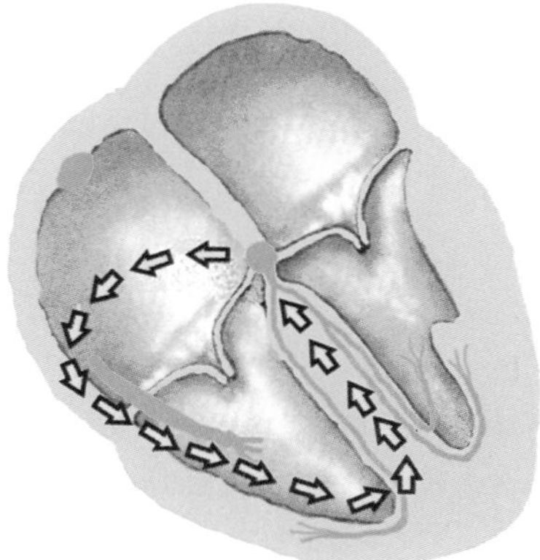

FIGURE 5.10. A rarer form of AVRT in which impulses travel down the bypass tract and then up the His-Purkinje system and AV node back to the atria. This pattern of impulse conduction is called antidromic conduction and results in wide QRS complexes occurring at a regular rate.

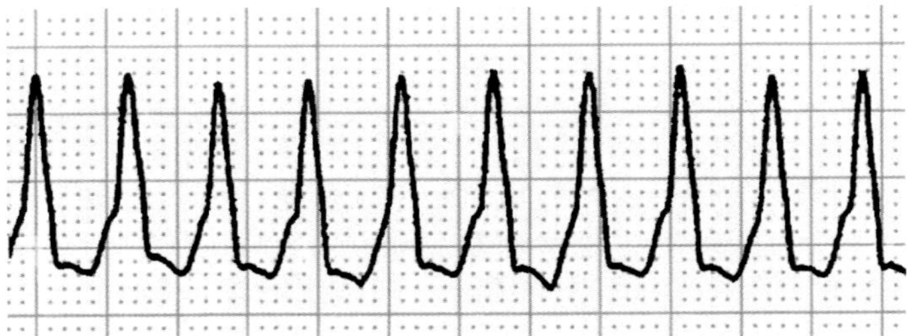

FIGURE 5.11. The wide complex regular rhythm produced by antidromic conduction in AVRT. Note this could easily be mistaken for monomorphic VT.

Like AVNRT, AVRT is due to a primary electrical problem with the heart, and is not associated with structural or ischemic heart disease. Also like AVNRT, the arrhythmia is often precipitated by a premature atrial contraction (PAC) or premature ventricular contraction (PVC).

The heart rate in patients who develop AVRT is most commonly in the range of 150–220 beats/min. Like AVNRT, the most common symptom is palpitations, although some persons may also experience lightheadedness, shortness of breath, or chest discomfort. Also like AVNRT, initial treatment is administration of medications that slow conduction through the AV node, which breaks the arrhythmia. These medicines include adenosine, beta blockers, and certain calcium channel blockers. Long-term treatment for many patients with WPW syndrome who develop arrhythmias is catheter ablation of the bypass tract.

CHAPTER 6

Tachyarrhythmias Originating in the Ventricles

Arrhythmias that originate in the ventricles, called "ventricular arrhythmias", are the most concerning tachyarrhythmias, as they can lead to hemodynamic collapse and death. We can again break down the common types of ventricular arrhythmias into one of three categories:

1. Ventricular tachycardia (VT)
2. Torsade de Pointes (a special type of ventricular tachycardia)
3. Ventricular fibrillation (VF)

Ventricular Tachycardia

Ventricular tachycardia (often referred to as "VT" or "V-tach") is a potentially fatal arrhythmia that originates and occurs in the ventricles (Figure 6.1). There are several basic mechanisms that can cause VT. One basic cause is that an area of tissue someplace in one of the ventricles starts to spontaneously depolarize at a fast rate and as you may remember is called "enhanced automaticity". The depolarization impulse generated then spreads throughout the ventricles, depolarizing the ventricles. The second basic mechanism that can cause VT is that depolarization impulse circles around and around part of the ventricle, resulting in a reentrant circuit. Such reentrant circuits can form around parts of the ventricles in which there is acute ischemia (such as an acute MI), where there is an old scar from a prior MI, or where there was a prior MI and an aneurysm has now formed.

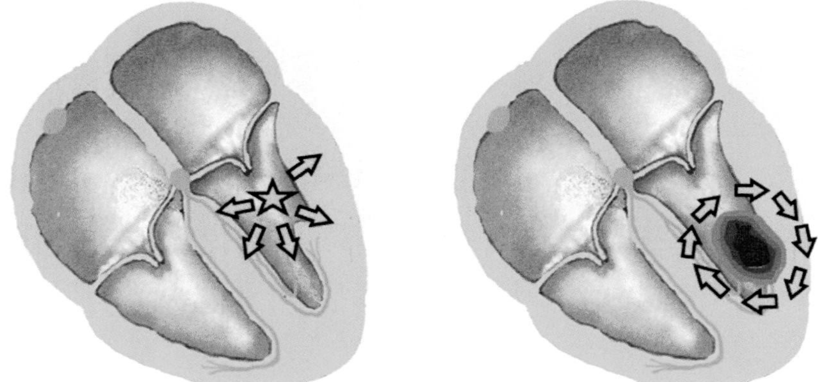

FIGURE 6.1. VT can be caused by enhanced automaticity (left) or by a reentrant circuit (right).

The risk of ventricular tachycardia is increased in patients with coronary artery disease, prior MI, cardiomyopathy, and/or depressed left ventricular ejection fraction. The heart rate with VT can be anywhere from the low 100s to 200 beats/min or more. While in some cases patients may experience only palpitations or lightheadedness, in other patients effective contractions of the ventricles are no longer present and the patient becomes pulseless. Stable VT, in which the patient has only minimal or mild symptoms, is usually treated with antiarrhythmic drugs or synchronized cardioversion. Pulseless VT is a medical emergency in which cardiac output is not sufficient to adequately perfuse the brain and other bodily tissues, and is treated with immediate defibrillation. We will discuss the treatment of VT further in the section on basic life support and advanced cardiac life support in Chapter 15.)

There are several other ways in which VT is classified. One way is classifying the VT based on its duration. "Non-sustained VT" is the term used if the arrhythmia lasts <30 seconds before self-terminating. "Sustained VT" is if the arrhythmia lasts >30 seconds.

Yet another way of classifying VT is based on its morphology. If all the wide QRS complexes look reasonably similar in shape, the

VT is called "monomorphic VT" (Figure 6.2). If the morphology of the QRS complexes notably varies, the arrhythmia is termed "polymorphic VT". While some patients who develop monomorphic VT are at least relatively stable, patients who develop polymorphic VT are usually unstable and may rapidly become pulseless. Polymorphic VT usually develops in patients with acute myocardial ischemia or in those with prolonged QT intervals (which comprises the repolarization phase of the heart) (Figures 6.3 and 6.4).

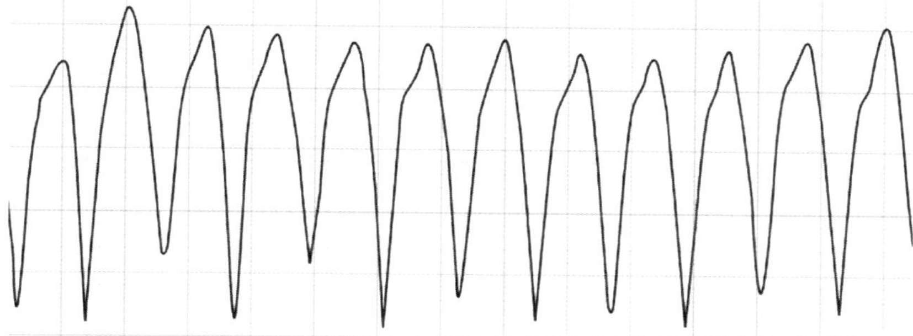

FIGURE 6.2. An example of monomorphic VT. All the QRS complexes look fairly similar in morphology.

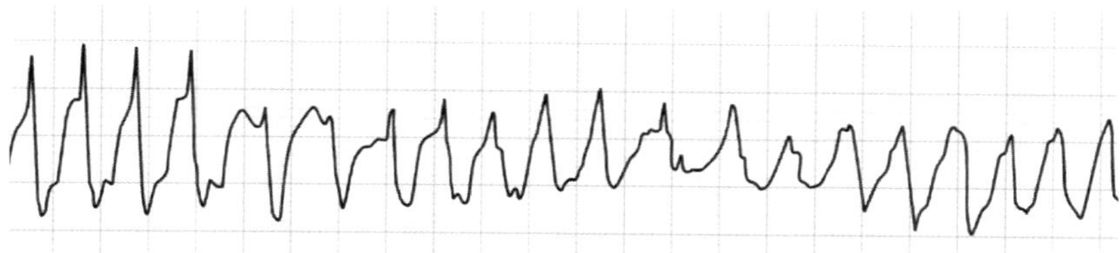

FIGURE 6.3. An example of polymorphic VT. There is marked variation in the QRS complex morphologies.

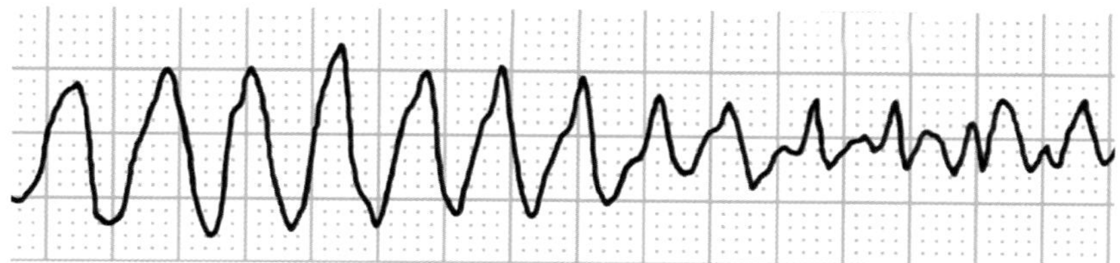

FIGURE 6.4. A second example of polymorphic VT. This is a critically important arrhythmia for you to be able to recognize.

Torsade de Pointes

A special type of polymorphic VT that occurs when the QT interval is prolonged is called "Torsade de Pointes". The QT interval can be congenitally abnormally prolonged or can be prolonged by drugs such as certain antiarrhythmic agents (such as procainamide, quinidine, sotalol, amiodarone, and ibutilide) or certain combinations of medicines. Torsade de Pointes is a French term that means "twisting of the points." In Torsade de Pointes, the axis of the QRS complex can be imagined to be rotating around a point, as shown in the ECG strip in Figure 6.5.

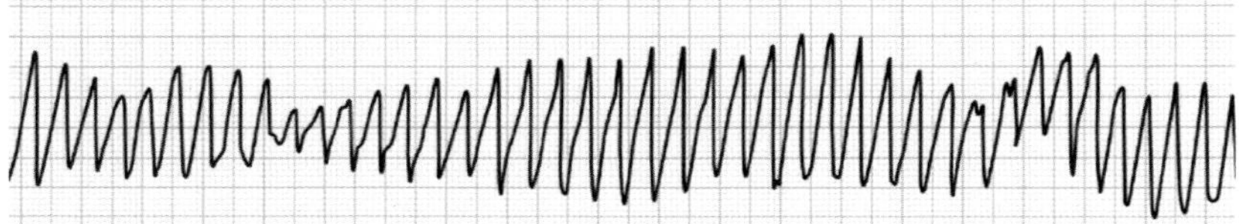

FIGURE 6.5. Torsade de Pointes. A special type of polymorphic ventricular tachycardia in which the imaginary axis of the QRS complexes seems to twist around a point.

Patients who develop Torsade de Pointes usually become hemodynamically unstable. The arrhythmia can quickly lead to death if not promptly treated with defibrillation.

Ventricular Fibrillation

Ventricular fibrillation (abbreviated as "VF" or "V-fib") is a state in which there is only disorganized electrical activity occurring in the ventricles. As there is no organized electric activity or ventricular contractions, the patient is pulseless and brain damage and death can rapidly ensue. VF is probably the most common cause of sudden death. Since in VF there is no organized depolarization of the ventricles, normal QRS complexes are not seen. Rather, the disorganized electrical activity is reflected on the ECG by smaller, somewhat random, deflections of the baseline, as shown in Figure 6.6.

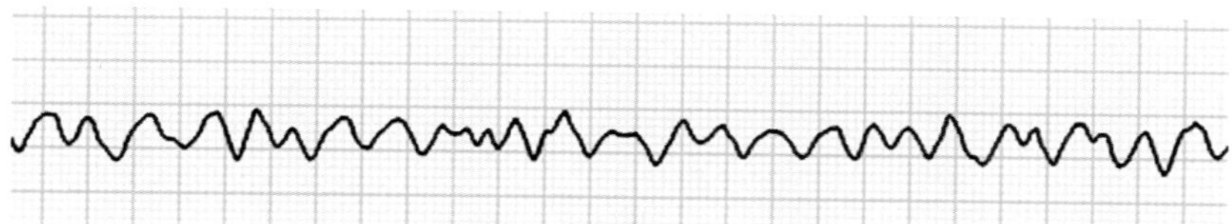

FIGURE 6.6. Ventricular fibrillation. No discrete QRS complexes are present.

VF most commonly occurs in patients with coronary artery disease and in many cases may be related to acute ischemia or acute MI. It also occurs in patients with depressed left ventricular ejection fraction and cardiomyopathies. VF is also associated with electrolyte abnormalities, such as hypokalemia. VF may result from untreated ventricular tachycardia, which may degenerate to VF. A second example of the ECG tracing of VF is shown in Figure 6.7.

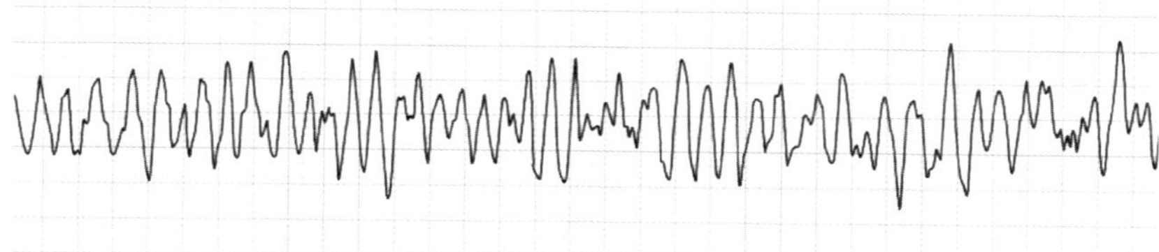

FIGURE 6.7. Another example of ventricular fibrillation, showing the disorganized electrical activity that occurs with this lethal arrhythmia.

The treatment of VF is immediate defibrillation. CPR should be administered while awaiting a defibrillator if a defibrillator is not immediately available. Treatment of VF is discussed further in Chapter 15.

CHAPTER 7

Diagnosing Tachyarrhythmias—General Approach

Now that we have discussed the various types of tachyarrhythmias, the next step is to discuss how we can diagnose the specific rhythm causing a tachyarrhythmia seen on an ECG or telemetry monitor. We will use a simple three-step process to help categorize and diagnose arrhythmias. The 3 simple steps, which we will discuss in more detail, are:

1. Determine if the QRS complexes seen in the arrhythmia are narrow or wide.
2. Determine if the QRS complexes are occurring at regular or irregular intervals.
3. Determine if there is any evidence of P waves or atrial activity present.

A narrow QRS complex is defined as a QRS complex that is <120 msec in width (< 3 little boxes in width on the ECG strip). A wide QRS complex is a QRS complex that is ≥120 msec in width (three or more little boxes in width on the ECG strip). Figure 7.1 shows examples of narrow and wide QRS complexes.

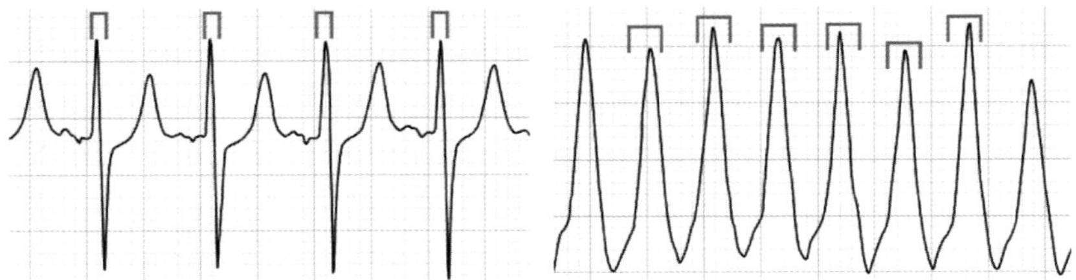

FIGURE 7.1. Narrow (left) and wide (right) QRS complexes.

By "regular" we mean that the QRS complexes are all occurring at regular intervals, like the ticking of a clock. In contrast, when the QRS complexes occur at irregular or varying intervals, like the sound of rain droplets falling, we say that the rhythm is "irregular". Figure 7.2 shows examples of QRS complexes that occur at regular intervals and QRS complexes that occur at irregular intervals

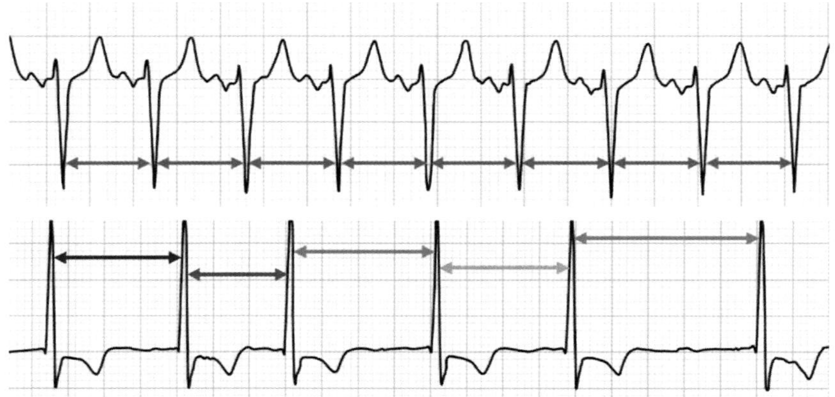

FIGURE 7.2. A regular rhythm (top), in which the QRS complexes occur at regular intervals, and an irregular rhythm (bottom), in which the intervals between QRS complexes vary.

Based on whether the QRS complexes are narrow or wide, and whether the QRS complexes are occurring at regular or irregular intervals, tachyarrhythmias are categorized in three basic categories:

1. Narrow complex regular tachycardias
2. Narrow complex irregular tachycardias
3. Wide complex tachycardias

Once we determine if the arrhythmia is a narrow complex regular tachycardia, a narrow complex irregular tachycardia, or a wide complex tachycardia, we determine the specific rhythm by looking for P waves or atrial activity.

In the following chapters, we will go through how this three-step method can be used to identify and diagnose specific tachyarrhythmias.

CHAPTER 8

Diagnosing Tachyarrhythmias—Narrow Complex Regular Tachycardia

There are six rhythms that can cause a narrow complex regular tachycardia:

- Sinus tachycardia
- Atrial tachycardia
- Atrial flutter
- Junctional tachycardia
- AV nodal reentrant tachycardia (AVNRT)
- AV reentrant tachycardia (AVRT)

We determine which of these rhythms causes the narrow complex tachycardia by looking for the presence (or absence) of any P waves or atrial activity before the QRS complexes. If there are normal looking P waves before each QRS, the rhythm is simply sinus tachycardia, as shown in Figure 8.1.

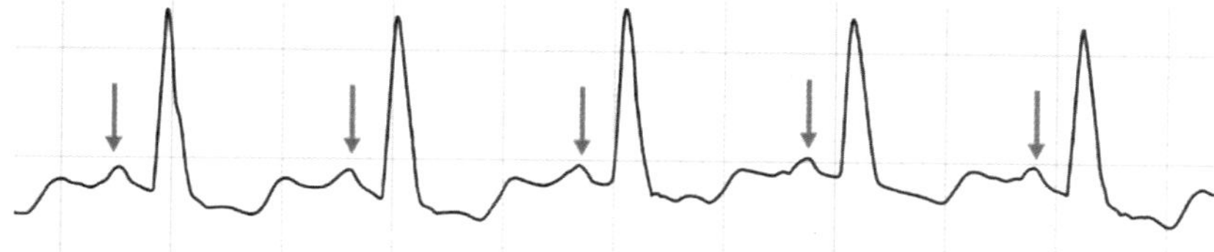

FIGURE 8.1. Sinus tachycardia. Normal looking P waves (arrows) are present before each QRS complex.

If there are abnormal appearing or inverted P waves before each QRS complex, then the rhythm is atrial tachycardia (Figure 8.2).

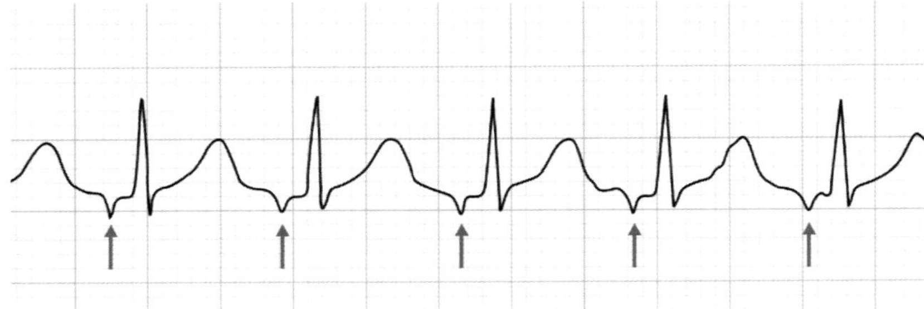

FIGURE 8.2. Atrial tachycardia. Abnormal-looking, inverted P waves (arrows) are present before each QRS complex.

If instead of discrete P waves, we see a sawtooth pattern of atrial activity with flutter waves, the rhythm is atrial flutter (Figure 8.3).

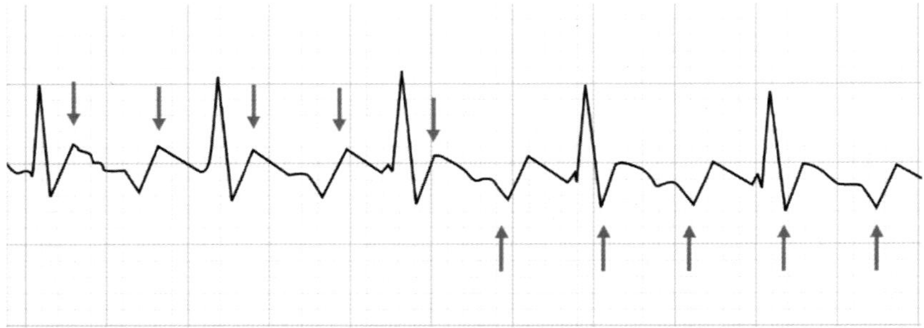

FIGURE 8.3. Atrial flutter. A sawtooth pattern of atrial activity, flutter waves, is present.

If we see neither P waves before the QRS complexes nor flutter waves, then the rhythm is either junctional tachycardia, AV nodal reentrant tachycardia (AVNRT) or AV reentrant tachycardia (AVRT). If the rhythm is at a rate of 100–120 beats/min, it is more likely than not the rhythm is junctional tachycardia, since AVNRT and AVRT usually result in a faster heart rate than this (Figure 8.4). If the rhythm is 140 beats/min or more, the rhythm is more likely to be AVNRT or AVRT than junctional tachycardia. It is usually impossible to determine for sure from the ECG whether the rhythm is AVNRT or AVRT. Statistically, AVNRT is much more common than AVRT, so in most cases the arrhythmia turns out to be due to AVNRT. However, if the patient has known WPW and a bypass tract, then the rhythm is more likely AVRT.

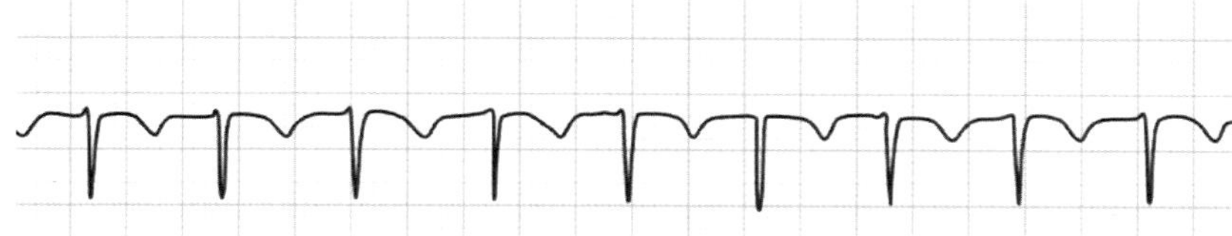

FIGURE 8.4. Junctional tachycardia. Regular narrow QRS complexes are present at a rate of 120 beats/min. No P waves are present.

In both AVNRT and AVRT, discrete P waves may not be visible. In fact, in 80% of cases of AVNRT, any retrograde P waves are hidden (buried) within the QRS complex and are thus not visible. However, if P waves occur after the QRS complexes are visible, this may help at least a little in deciding whether the rhythm is more likely AVNRT or AVRT. If retrograde P waves are seen at the end of the QRS complex or immediately after the QRS complex, this may make it a little more likely the rhythm is AVNRT, whereas if retrograde P waves are seen a discrete distance from the QRS complexes, this may make it a little more likely the rhythm is AVRT. The rhythm strips in Figures 8.5–8.7 illustrate this concept. It should be noted, however, that there are exceptions to this generalization, and the distance of the retrograde P waves from the QRS complexes cannot be used to definitively decide whether the rhythm is AVNRT or AVRT.

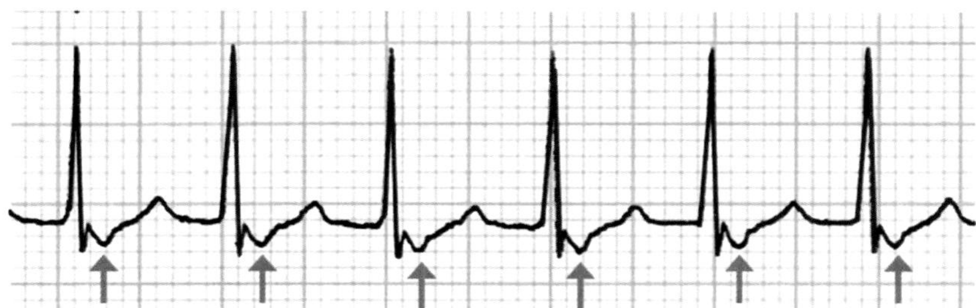

FIGURE 8.5. In this narrow complex regular tachycardia, retrograde P waves (arrows) are visible immediately after the QRS complexes, making the more likely diagnosis AVNRT.

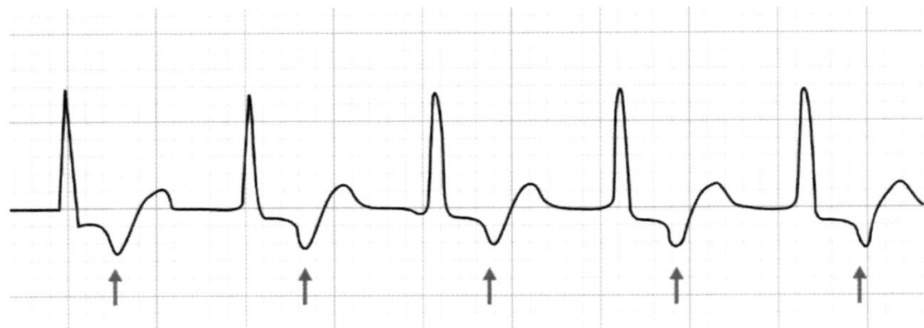

FIGURE 8.6. In this narrow complex regular tachycardia, retrograde P waves (arrows) are visible a notable distance after the QRS complexes, in the ST segment, making it a little more likely that this arrhythmia is AVRT and not AVNRT.

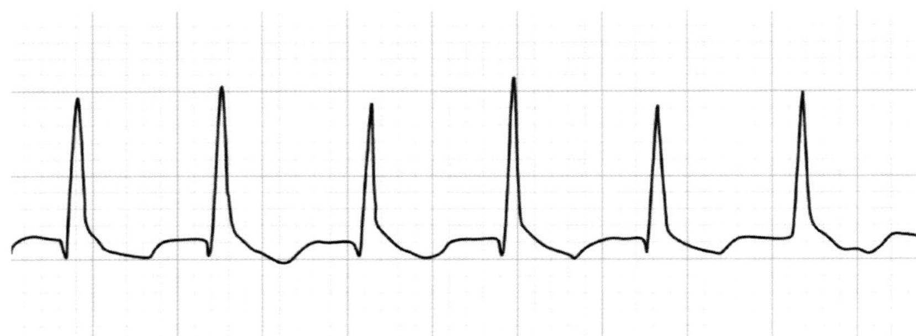

FIGURE 8.7. In this narrow complex regular tachycardia no P waves or flutter waves are visible before or after the QRS complexes. The rate of 180 beats/min makes this arrhythmia too fast to be junctional tachycardia, and it is either AVNRT or AVRT.

In summary, once we determine that the QRS complexes are narrow and occur at regular intervals, to determine the rhythm we look for P waves or atrial activity:

- Normal P waves before each QRS complex → sinus tachycardia
- Abnormal or inverted P waves before each QRS complex → atrial tachycardia
- Flutter waves → atrial flutter

- No P waves or retrograde P waves after the QRS complexes and at a rate of approximately 100–120 bpm → junctional tachycardia
- No P waves or retrograde P waves after the QRS complexes and at a rate of approximately ≥140 bpm → AVNRT or AVRT

CHAPTER 9

Diagnosing Tachyarrhythmias—Narrow Complex Irregular Tachycardia

There are three rhythms that can cause a narrow complex irregular tachycardia:

1. Multifocal atrial tachycardia (MAT)
2. Atrial flutter with variable conduction
3. Atrial fibrillation

As we did with the narrow complex regular tachycardias, to determine the cause of a narrow complex irregular tachycardia we look for P waves or atrial activity before the QRS complexes. If there are P waves of differing morphologies before each QRS complex, then the rhythm is MAT (Figure 9.1).

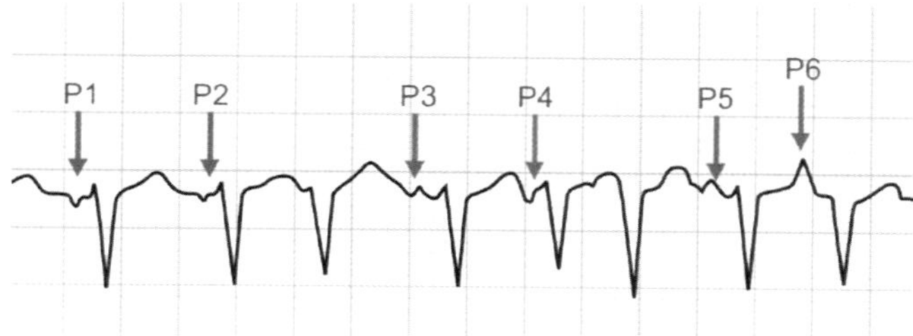

FIGURE 9.1. Multifocal Atrial Tachycardia (MAT. There are P waves of differing morphology before each QRS complex. In this example, at least six different P wave morphologies are present.

In the rhythm strip in Figure 9.2, flutter waves are clearly visible, making the diagnosis of atrial flutter. Previously, we have seen an example of atrial flutter in which there are two flutter waves for each QRS complex, which results from 2:1 conduction down the AV node. Occasionally, in atrial flutter we see a variable conduction or variable block of depolarization impulses down the AV node. For instance, there may be 2:1 conduction for a couple beats, then 1:1 conduction for a beat, then 3:1 conduction for several beats, then more 2:1 conduction. In such cases, instead of QRS complexes occurring at regular intervals, the QRS complexes occur at irregular intervals.

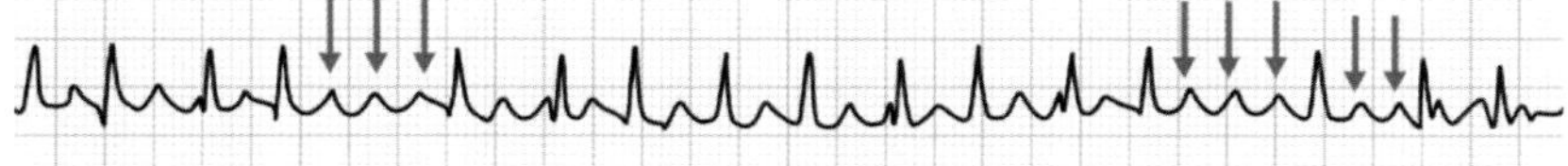

FIGURE 9.2. Atrial flutter with variable block. There is a varying ratio of flutter waves to QRS complexes, resulting in an irregular rhythm. When there is 2:1 conduction, many of the flutter waves are not visible, buried in the QRS complexes. However, when there are periods of 3:1 or 4:1 conduction, the flutter waves (arrows) are more visible.

In the example of the following narrow complex irregular rhythm, there are no P waves or ECG signs of organized atrial activity present. The rhythm is therefore atrial fibrillation (Figure 9.3). Notice that in atrial fibrillation there can be some modest irregular and random deflections of the ECG baseline, but these deflections should not be mistaken for P waves or flutter waves.

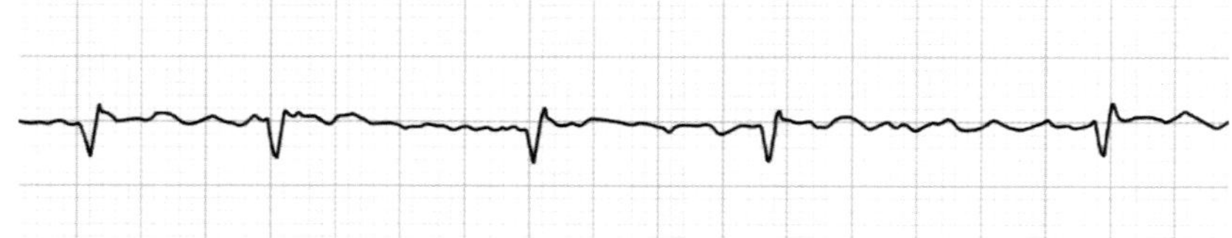

FIGURE 9.3. Atrial fibrillation. There are no P waves or flutter waves present, only modest random and irregular deflections of the ECG baseline.

In summary, once we determine that the QRS complexes are narrow and occur at irregular intervals, we look for the presence of

P waves or atrial activity to determine which of the three possible rhythms are causing the arrhythmia:

1. Multiple P waves of differing morphology before each QRS complex → Multifocal atrial tachycardia (MAT)
2. Flutter waves → atrial flutter
3. No P waves or organized atrial activity → atrial fibrillation

CHAPTER 10

Diagnosing Tachyarrhythmias—Wide Complex Tachycardia

There are two basic causes of a wide complex tachycardia:

- Any type of supraventricular tachycardia (SVT) in which there is bundle branch block causing the QRS complex to be wide
- Ventricular tachycardia (VT)

We need to take a minute to explain what we mean by a supraventricular tachycardia (SVT) with bundle branch block (BBB). Remember that by SVT, we mean any tachyarrhythmia that does not originate in the ventricles. Thus, SVT includes all the arrhythmias we have discussed other than ventricular tachycardia. Both a right bundle branch block (RBBB) and a left bundle branch block (LBBB) result in a wide QRS complex. Therefore, any combination of SVT and BBB results in a wide complex tachycardia appearing on the ECG. Note that for the purposes of this discussion we consider sinus tachycardia in the same category as supraventricular tachycardias, so sinus tachycardia with a BBB also produces a wide complex tachycardia.

To diagnose the cause of a wide complex tachycardia, we again use our three-step process, modifying it slightly for wide complex tachycardias:

1. Determine if the QRS complexes are narrow or wide.
2. Determine if the QRS complexes are perfectly regular or slightly irregular.

3. Determine if P waves or evidence of atrial activity are present before each QRS complex, or if there is evidence of P wave (or AV) dissociation.

Step 1 is a "give me" in golf vernacular, since we have already determined that the QRS complexes are wide.

Step 2 is to determine if the QRS complexes are perfectly regular or slightly irregular. While a SVT with BBB will usually appear perfectly regular, both in terms of QRS morphology and the RR interval (which is the distance between QRS complexes) — what my arrhythmia mentor termed the "boringly regular QRS complexes of a SVT" — VT often appears slightly irregular, both in terms of the QRS morphology itself, and the RR interval. Below is an example of a SVT with BBB. Each QRS complex looks exactly like the others, and the RR intervals are exactly the same. As my arrhythmia mentor described it, these QRS complexes are the boringly regular wide QRS complexes seen in an SVT (Figure 10.1).

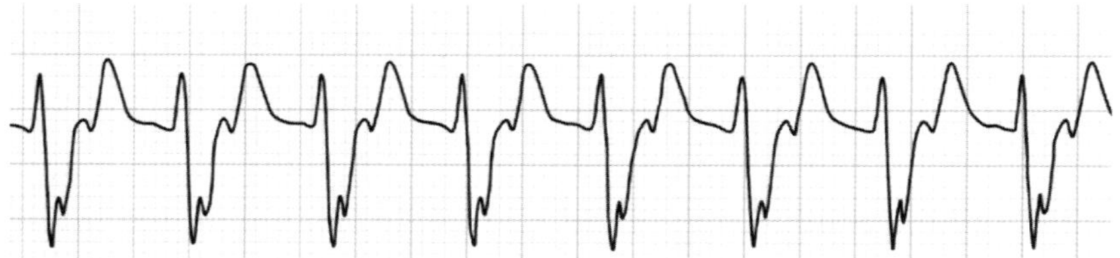

FIGURE 10.1. The boringly regular wide QRS complexes seen in an SVT with bundle branch block.

In contrast, in Figure 10.2's example of monomorphic VT, there is still a slight variation in the QRS morphologies and the RR intervals.

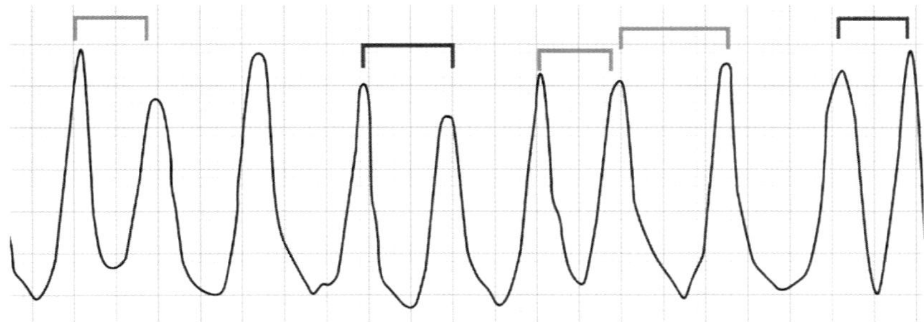

FIGURE 10.2. In this example of monomorphic VT, the QRS intervals are slightly irregular in morphology and the RR intervals (brackets) are also slightly irregular.

Perfectly regular wide complex tachycardias are *usually* SVT with BBB, although occasionally a monomorphic VT may look almost perfectly regular. Therefore, the presence of a perfectly regular wide complex tachycardia makes us suspect it is likely due to an SVT with BBB, but we cannot say for certain this is the case. In contrast, a wide complex tachycardia that is slightly irregular is usually VT (Figure 10.3).

Heartman's Clinical Pearl

A rare exception to the above rule is occasionally seen in patients with Wolff-Parkinson-White (WPW) syndrome who develop atrial fibrillation. Patients with WPW who develop atrial fibrillation have an unusual ECG that shows an irregular rhythm and QRS complexes of varying width. This is because some of the impulses that reach and depolarize the ventricle travel down the AV node and His-Purkinje system, resulting in narrow QRS complexes, while some other impulses that depolarize the ventricle travel down the bypass tract, resulting in wide QRS complexes. Sometimes, impulses traveling down the AV node and His-Purkinje system and impulses traveling down the bypass tract arrive in the ventricle at the same time, resulting in a QRS impulse that is a hybrid of a narrow QRS complex and a wide QRS complex. The resulting rhythm strip of a patient with WPW who developed atrial fibrillation is shown below, and is essentially a montage of narrow QRS complexes, wide QRS complexes, and QRS complexes of intermediate width.

Patients who develop this arrhythmia should not be treated with medications that slow conduction down the AV node, as this may—somewhat paradoxically—lead to an increase in heart rate as more impulses travel down the bypass tract and depolarize the ventricles, which can lead the patient to develop ventricular fibrillation

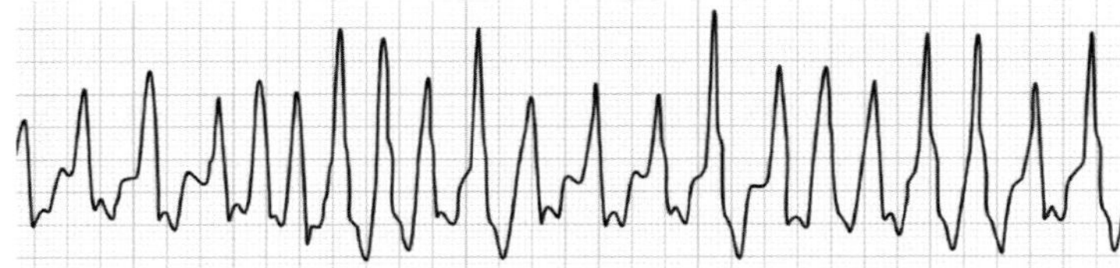

FIGURE 10.3. An example of atrial fibrillation in a patient with WPW. There is marked variation in the QRS complex morphologies and RR intervals.

A second trick to help distinguish SVT with BBB from VT is to look for P waves or organized atrial activity. If we see P waves or flutter waves before each QRS complex, then we know the rhythm must be some type of SVT (or sinus tachycardia) with BBB. For example, in Figure 10.4, rhythm strip P waves (arrows) can be seen before each wide QRS complex. The rhythm is thus sinus tachycardia.

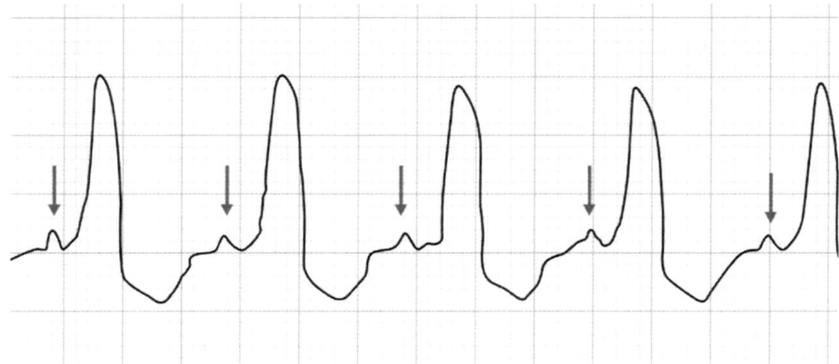

FIGURE 10.4. Sinus tachycardia with LBBB. Normal looking P waves (arrows) are present before each QRS complex.

We also look for P waves any place in the ECG to see if something called “P wave dissociation” is present. P wave dissociation (interchangeably called “AV dissociation”) is a phenomenon that occurs in some patients who develop VT. In such patients, VT develops in the ventricle, depolarizing the ventricle. While this depolarization is occurring in the ventricles, at the same time the SA node up in the right atrium may continue to generate impulses which depolarize the atria. Depolarization of the atria and the ventricles occurs independently of each other, hence the term AV dissociation. This phenomenon is illustrated in the Figure 10.5.

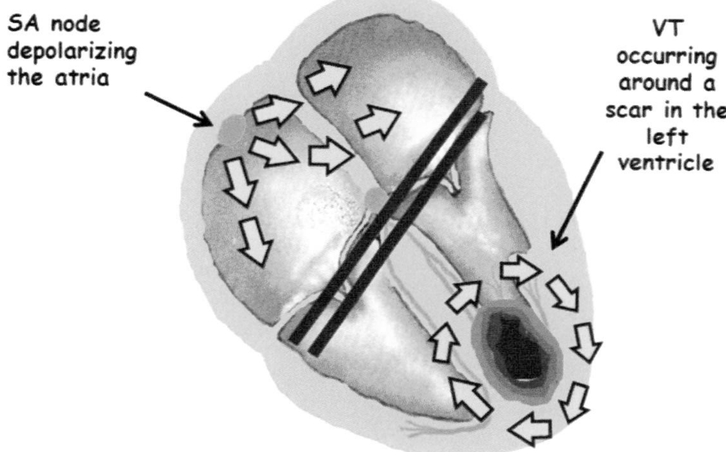

FIGURE 10.5. P wave dissociation (also called AV dissociation) occurring during ventricular tachycardia. The atria and ventricles depolarize independent of each other.

On the ECG in Figure 10.6, we see the fast and wide QRS complexes of VT. We also may see an occasional P wave, caused by depolarization of the atria. Since the atria and the ventricles are depolarizing at different rates, there is no relationship seen between the P waves and the QRS complexes, hence the terms “P wave dissociation” or “AV dissociation” (the terms are used interchangeably). These dissociated P waves may be seen any place on the ECG, including in the ST or T waves. The finding on the ECG of P wave dissociation (AV dissociation) is extremely helpful in making the diagnosis of the arrhythmia, since the finding of P wave dissociation almost always means the wide complex arrhythmia is due to VT (Figures 10.6–10.8).

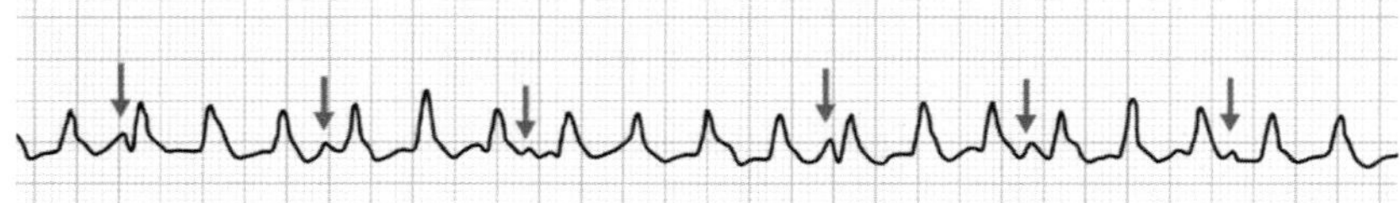

FIGURE 10.6. An example of P wave dissociation (AV dissociation) occurring in a patient with VT. There is no relationship between the P waves (arrows) and the QRS complexes.

Heartman's Clinical Pearl

For the purposes of simplicity, we discussed that a wide complex tachycardia can basically be caused by one of two arrhythmias, either an SVT with bundle branch block or ventricular tachycardia. You may remember, however, that earlier in the book we discussed that in a small percentage (5%–10%) of cases of AVRT, the impulse travels down the bypass tract, into the ventricle, then up the His-Purkinje system and AV node, and into the atria. When this type of reentrant circuit occurs (which we discussed is called "antidromic conduction"), the resulting QRS complexes are wide (as depolarization across the ventricle occurs slowly). Thus, technically, there are three causes of a wide complex tachycardia:

1. *SVT with bundle branch block*
2. *ARVT with antidromic conduction*
3. *VT*

As this is only a rare cause of a wide complex tachycardia, do not worry if you do not understand this or do not want to spend time memorizing this. This is important at the level of a cardiologist, but not critical to someone first learning arrhythmia diagnosis and treatment.

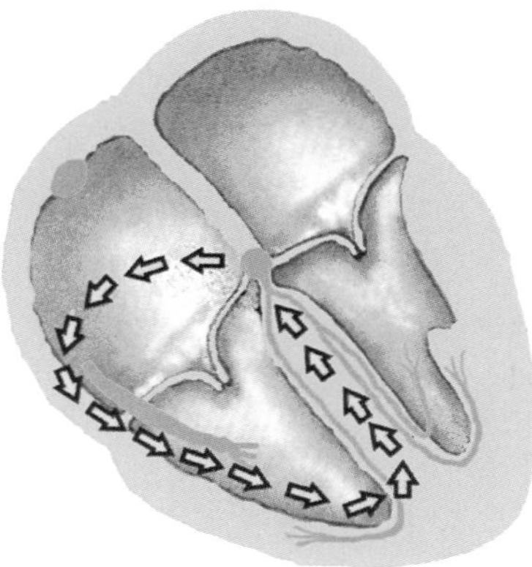

FIGURE 10.7. A rare form of AVRT in which impulses travel down the bypass tract, across the ventricles, and then up the His-Purkinje system and AV node back to the atria. This pattern of impulse conduction, called "antidromic conduction", results in wide QRS complexes occurring at regular intervals.

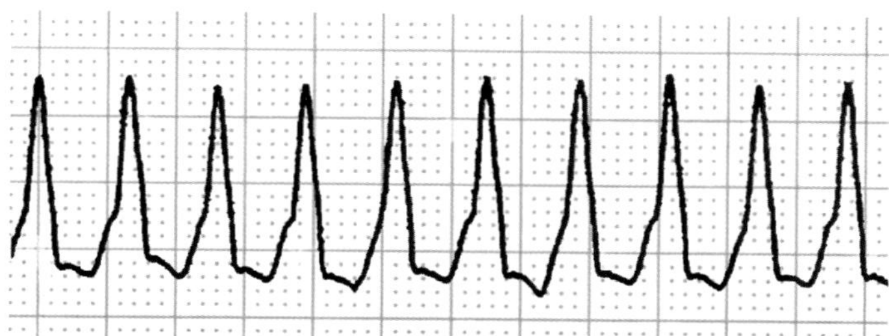

FIGURE 10.8. The wide QRS complexes occurring at regular intervals with antidromic AVRT.

In summary, there are a couple of tricks we can use to help distinguish a rhythm caused by SVT with BBB from a rhythm due to VT:

1. Look to see if the QRS complexes are perfectly regular or slightly irregular. If the QRS morphologies and RR intervals are all perfectly the same, then this suggests the rhythm is likely SVT with BBB. If there is slight (or more) variation in the QRS morphologies and RR intervals, then the rhythm is likely VT.

2. Look for P waves or organized atrial activity. If there are P waves before each QRS complex, or flutter waves present, then the rhythm is SVT with BBB. If there is P wave dissociation (AV dissociation), then the rhythm is VT.

CHAPTER 11

Bradyarrhythmias and Heart Block

In this chapter, we will discuss and review the heart rhythms that can cause a bradyarrhythmia. Bradycardia is defined as a heart rate of <60 beats/min. A bradyarrhythmia is therefore any abnormal rhythm that results in a heart rate of <60 beats/min. While some cases of bradyarrhythmia are relatively benign, some can be life threatening, so it is important to be able to identify the cause of the bradyarrhythmia.

Sinus Bradycardia

The normal rate of depolarization of the SA node is 60–100 beats/min. When the SA node depolarizes at <60 beats/min, and the ventricle is depolarized at <60 beats/min, the resulting rhythm is sinus bradycardia, as shown in Figure 11.1.

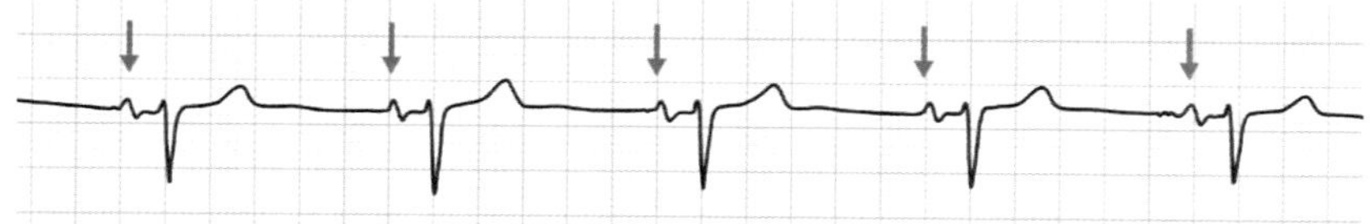

FIGURE 11.1. Sinus bradycardia. A P wave is present before each QRS complex. The heart rate is 50 beats/min.

Numerous conditions and factors can lead to a sinus bradycardia. Sinus bradycardia can also be seen in well-conditioned athletes or simply as a normal variant in otherwise healthy persons. Some of the most important causes are listed in Table 11.1.

Unless the heart rate is <40–50 beats/min or so, patients are rarely symptomatic. In the rare patient who requires treatment for sinus bradycardia, the first step is to address any potential cause, such as discontinuing drugs that slow depolarization of the SA node (such as beta blockers or the calcium channel blockers verapamil and diltiazem). In most cases of severely symptomatic bradycardia, acute treatment involves administration of atropine. Temporary transcutaneous pacing is also employed when available in severely symptomatic patients. The acute treatment of symptomatic bradycardia is discussed more in Chapter 15. Long-term treatment of patients with symptomatic bradycardia is pacemaker implantation.

TABLE 11.1. Causes of sinus bradycardia

• Medications that slow depolarization of the SA node (eg, beta blockers, the calcium channel blockers verapamil and diltiazem, digoxin, and antiarrhythmic agents such as amiodarone)
• Intrinsic SA nodal disease (sick sinus syndrome, such as can occur in elderly patients)
• Hypothyroidism
• Electrolyte abnormalities (eg, severe hyperkalemia)
• Increased vagal tone (such as with an acute inferior wall MI, vasovagal reaction, or as seen in high endurance athletes)
• Brain injury (stroke or trauma),
• Hypoxemia (low oxygen levels in the blood)

Junctional Rhythms

As we have discussed previously, the tissue of the SA node is able to spontaneously depolarize and act as the pacemaker of the heart. The lower part of the AV node is itself also able to spontaneously depolarize, similar to how the SA node spontaneously depolarizes. Since the normal rate of SA node depolarization (60–100 beats/min) is faster than the rate that the lower part of the AV node spontaneously depolarizes (40–60 beats/min), the SA node usually acts as the pacemaker of the heart. If, however, for some reason the SA node either depolarizes at a very slow rate or stops spontaneously depolarizing completely, this lower part of the AV node may take over as the pacemaker of the heart. When the AV node acts as the pacemaker of the heart, the rhythm is referred to as a "junctional rhythm" since it originates near the junction of the atria and the ventricles (where the lower part of the AV node is located).

The impulses generated by spontaneous depolarizations of the AV node normally travel down the His-Purkinje system into the ventricles, depolarizing the ventricles in the normal manner; thus, the QRS complexes in a junctional rhythm are narrow. Since the usual rate of spontaneous depolarization of the AV node is 40–60 beats/min, the ECG shows narrow QRS complexes usually at a rate of 40–60 beats/min. Since the AV node depolarizes at a regular rate, the resulting QRS impulses occur at regular intervals. In a junctional rhythm, depolarization of the SA node is no longer occurring; thus, normal P waves are usually not seen preceding each QRS complex, as in the ECG shown in Figure 11.2.

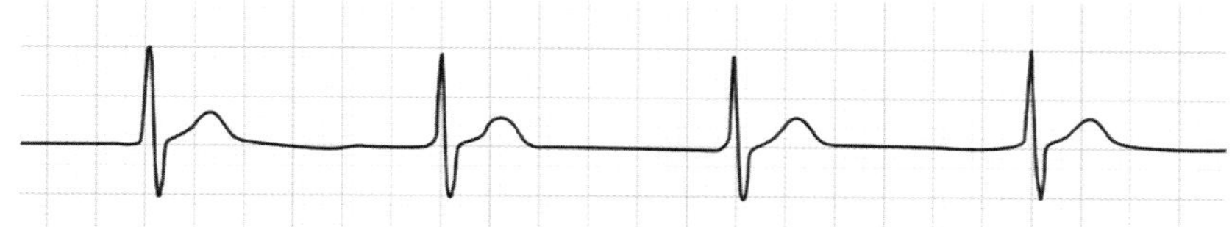

FIGURE 11.2. Junctional rhythm. There are narrow QRS complexes at a rate of 50 beats/min. No P waves are present before the QRS complexes.

While in most cases of junctional rhythm P waves are not present, in some cases P waves may be seen immediately before the QRS complexes. This can occur when the depolarization impulse generated by spontaneous depolarization of the AV node travels not only down into the ventricle but also "upward" into the atria, depolarization the atria from bottom to top. In such cases in which spontaneous depolarization of the AV nodal tissue leads to depolarization of the atria and the ventricles, depolarization of the atria and ventricles occur at almost the same time. When this occurs, an often "inverted" P wave may be seen immediately before the QRS complexes, as is shown in Figure 11.3. Note that the visible

P wave is very close to the QRS complex. Do not mistake this for sinus rhythm, in which we expect to see P waves a discrete distance (usually at least 120 msec or three "small boxes") before the QRS complexes.

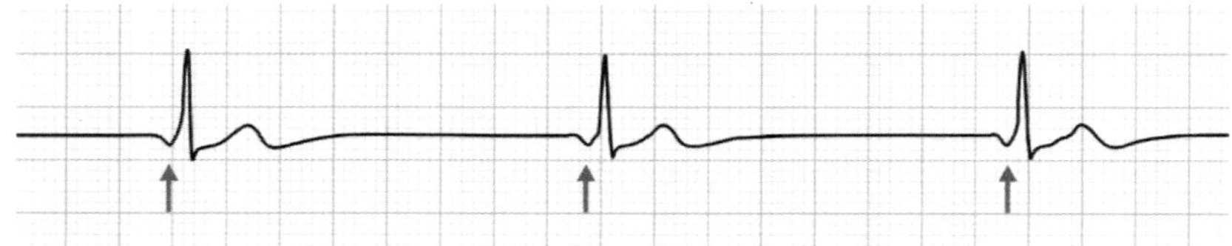

FIGURE 11.3. Junctional rhythm. In this example, retrograde, inverted P waves (arrows) are visible just before the QRS complexes.

Many persons who develop a junctional rhythm may be asymptomatic. In some, because of the relatively slow heart rate, dizziness, lightheadedness, presyncope (the sensation of being about to pass out), mild shortness of breath, fatigue, or decreased exercise ability may develop. Most patients who develop junctional rhythm require no specific acute treatment. Rather, management of such persons usually involves determining why they developed the junctional rhythm.

First-Degree Heart Block

In patients with first-degree heart block, each impulse generated by the SA node depolarizing is conducted down the AV node and His-Purkinje system to the ventricles, but conduction through the AV node down into the ventricles is slower than normal. This is reflected in the ECG in that each P wave is followed by a QRS complex, but the PR interval (the distance between the beginning of the P wave and the beginning of the QRS interval) is prolonged. By definition, first-degree heart block is when the PR interval is >200 msec (>5 small boxes on the ECG). First-degree heart block in itself does not result in bradycardia. First-degree heart block can be caused by medications that slow conduction through the AV node (eg, beta blockers, certain calcium channel blockers, digoxin, or antiarrhythmic agents such as amiodarone), increased vagal tone, or intrinsic disease of the AV node (which can occur with normal aging). Figure 11.4 shows an example of sinus rhythm with first-degree heart block.

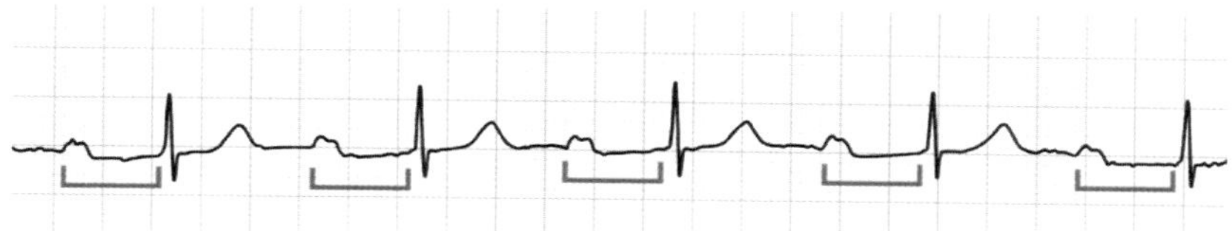

FIGURE 11.4. First-degree heart block, with a prolonged PR interval (brackets). The PR interval is >200 msec (5 small boxes).

Mobitz Type I Second-Degree Heart Block (Wenkebach)

Second-degree heart block is when some depolarization impulses generated by depolarization of the SA node are not conducted through the AV node into the ventricle. This results in an ECG in which not all P waves are followed by a QRS complex. When this occurs, we say that there are some "non-conducted impulses", "non-conducted P waves", or "non-conducted beats" present on the ECG. There are two types of second-degree heart block: Mobitz type I and Mobitz type II. First, we'll discuss Mobitz type I second-degree heart block.

Mobitz type I second-degree heart block is usually simply called "Wenkebach", and we will use that term here (Heartman explains this name in his next clinical pearl). In patients with Wenkebach, the ECG shows regularly occurring P waves, but the PR interval progressively increases, until there is a non-conducted P wave (a P wave not followed by a QRS complex). What occurs in the conduction system is that the time it takes the impulse generated by the SA node to travel through the AV node gets progressively longer and longer until one impulse generated by the SA node simply does not make it down the AV node to the ventricle. This results in a non-conducted P wave. Afterwards, the process begins again, with longer and longer PR intervals until another non-conducted P wave occurs. The ECG tracing in Wenkebach is shown in Figure 11.5.

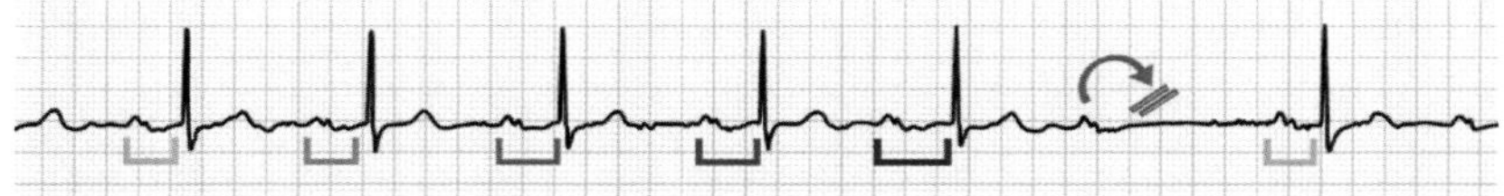

FIGURE 11.5. Wenkebach. The PR intervals progressively increase until there is a non-conducted P wave or "dropped beat". The brackets show the increasing PR intervals.

Wenkebach often occurs in persons with increased vagal tone, as vagal tone modulates conduction through the AV node. If it also sometimes seen in older patients. Wenkebach may or may not lead to bradycardia, depending on the rate of SA node depolarization and the ratio of conducted beats to non-conducted beats. Wenkebach is often incidentally noted on the telemetry monitor in hospitalized patients who are sleeping, as vagal tone increases during sleep. In itself, Wenkebach rarely causes the patient any symptoms and is a relatively benign rhythm. Although over time the patient may develop other conduction abnormalities, the presence of Wenkebach does not require any specific treatment, and is not an indication for pacemaker implantation.

Heartman's Clinical Pearl

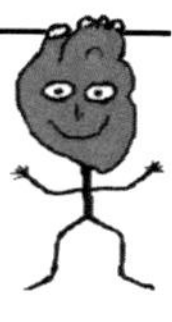

Fun fact. "Wenkebach" is not a made-up name. It is the rhythm described in 1899 by the Dutch cardiologist Karel Frederik Wenkebach, which now bears his name (Figure 11.6).

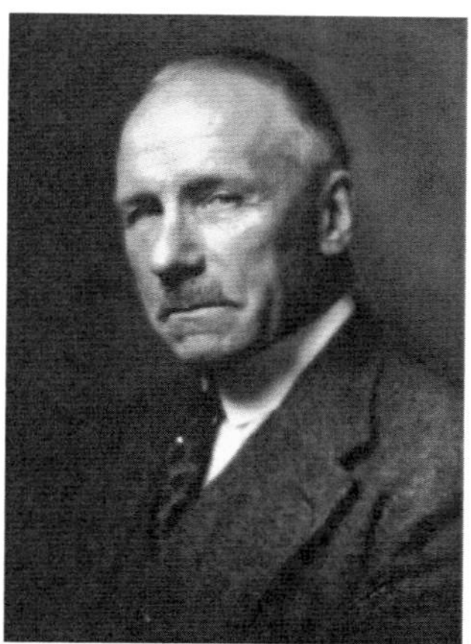

FIGURE 11.6. Karel Frederik Wenkebach. Image from Wikidata.

Mobitz Type II Second-Degree Heart Block

In Mobitz type II second-degree heart block, there are one or more P waves, each followed by a QRS complex, and then a non-conducted P wave (often called a "dropped beat") in which there is a P wave which is not followed by a QRS complex (Figure 11.7). In contrast to Wenkebach, in which the PR interval gradually increases until there is a non-conducted P wave, in Mobitz type II heart block the PR interval is constant, and the non-conducted P wave occurs "out of the blue" with no forewarning (Figure 11.8).

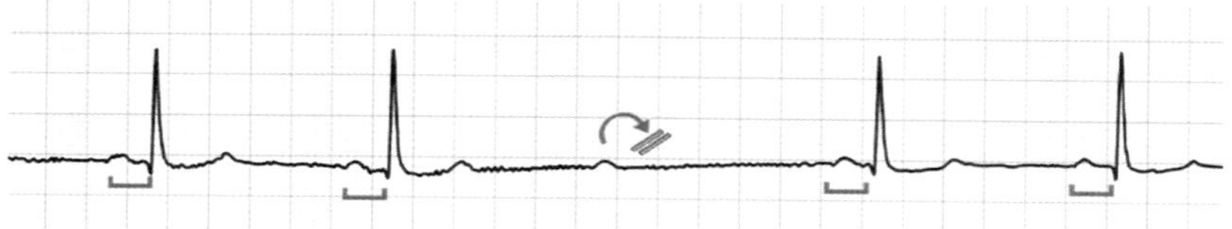

FIGURE 11.7. Mobitz type II heart block. The PR interval is constant until a non-conducted P wave abruptly occurs.

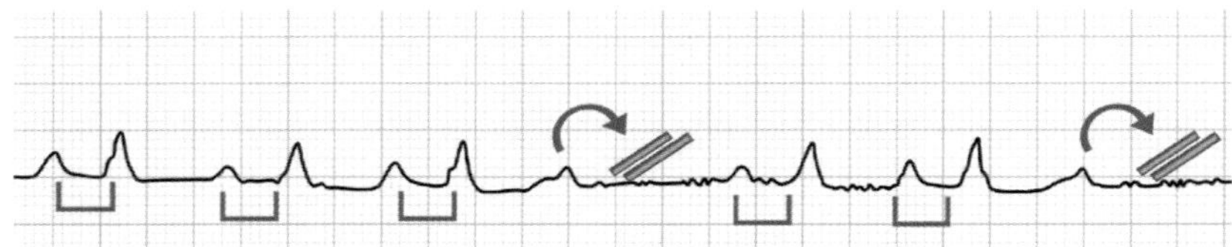

FIGURE 11.8. A second example of Mobitz type II heart block. The PR interval is constant until a non-conducted P wave abruptly occurs. The non-conducted P waves in this second example are present at the end of the T waves (look carefully!).

Like Wenkebach, Mobitz type II heart block may or may not lead to bradycardia, depending on the rate of SA node depolarization and the ratio of conducted to non-conducted P waves. Mobitz type II heart block may be due to progressive intrinsic disease within the AV node or acute MI. It is a concerning rhythm, and can progress to complete heart block. Therefore, such patients are hospitalized, placed on telemetry monitoring, and often have either transcutaneous pacing pads placed or a temporary transvenous pacing wire inserted. Permanent pacemaker implantation is usually expeditiously performed in such patients.

Third-Degree (Complete) Heart Block

Third-degree heart block, which is more commonly referred to as "complete heart block", occurs when no P waves are conducted through the AV node down to the ventricle. In such cases, one of three things can occur:

1. A junctional escape rhythm
2. A ventricular escape rhythm
3. Asystole (no heartbeat)

As we discussed previously, the lower part of the AV node is itself able to spontaneously depolarize, similar to how the SA node spontaneously depolarizes. If there is complete heart block, this lower part of the AV node may take over as the pacemaker of the heart. In cases of complete heart block, when the AV node takes over as the pacemaker of the heart the rhythm is referred to as a "junctional escape rhythm". These junctional rhythms consist of narrow QRS complexes at a rate usually of 40–60 beats/min. Since the SA node continues to spontaneously depolarize and depolarize the atria, P waves are seen on the ECG. Since, however, there is complete heart block present, the P waves are not followed by QRS complexes, but rather seem to "march through" the QRS complexes that occur as a result of the junctional escape rhythm. This is illustrated on the rhythm strip shown in Figure 11.9.

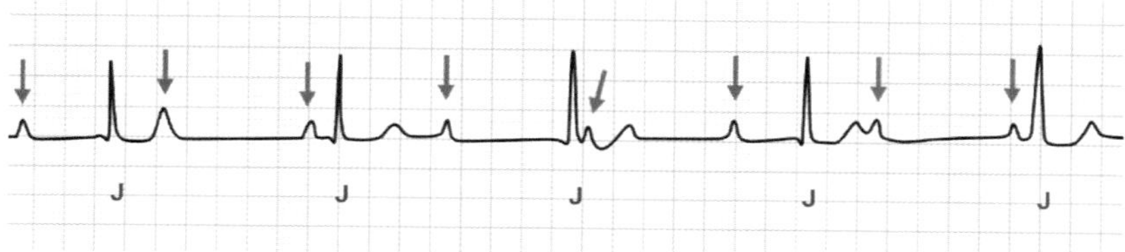

FIGURE 11.9. Complete heart block with a junctional escape rhythm. The P waves (arrows) are not conducted and there is a narrow QRS complex junctional escape rhythm (J).

Some myocardial cells (myocytes) located in the ventricles are also occasionally able to spontaneously depolarize. If there is complete heart block and there is no junctional escape rhythm, then these myocytes may assume the role of pacemaker of the heart. When there is complete heart block and cells in the ventricle begin to spontaneously depolarize, the rhythm is called a "ventricular escape rhythm". The rate of spontaneous depolarization of ventricular cells is usually 30–40 beats/min. Since in such cases depolarization of the heart begins in the ventricles, depolarization impulses have to spread cell to cell, instead of using the much faster His-Purkinje system to spread the depolarization impulse. This results in a wide QRS complex. Therefore, in patients with complete heart block and a ventricular escape rhythm, there are usually wide QRS complexes at a rate of 30–40 beats/min. An example of complete heart block with a ventricular escape rhythm is shown in the ECG tracing in Figure 11.10.

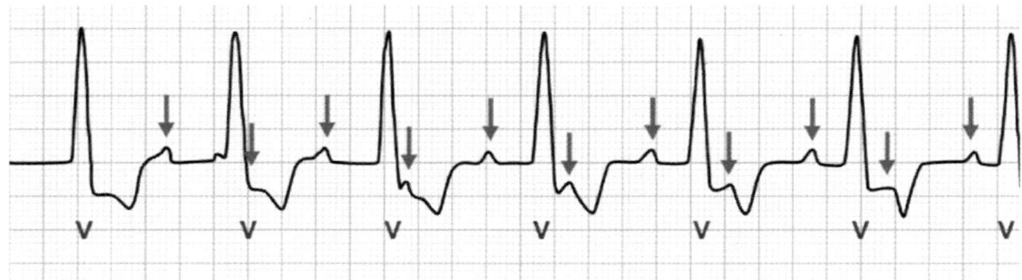

FIGURE 11.10. Complete heart block with a ventricular escape rhythm. The P waves (arrows) are not conducted and appear to march through the QRS complexes. The wide QRS complexes (V) are ventricular beats due to a ventricular escape rhythm.

The third thing that can occur when there is complete heart block is that there is complete heart block with neither a junctional escape rhythm nor a ventricular escape rhythm. In such cases, there is asystole and imminent death (Figure 11.11).

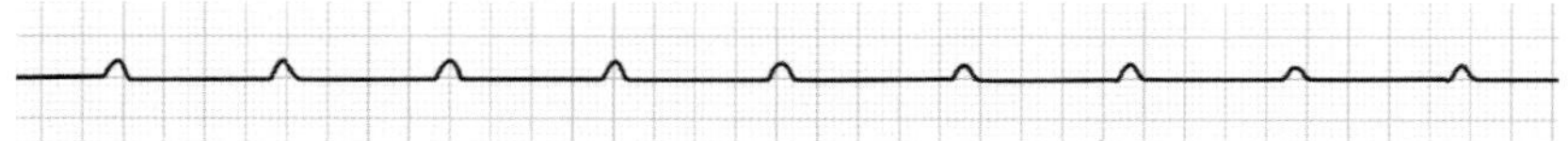

FIGURE 11.11. Complete heart block with asystole. Only P waves are visible and no QRS complexes are present. There is neither a junctional nor ventricular escape rhythm.

Causes of complete heart block include medication effects or frank overdose (eg, beta blockers, calcium channel blockers, digoxin, or antiarrhythmic agents), progressive intrinsic disease of the AV node, and acute MI.

Complete heart block is always an indication for admission, telemetry monitoring, and intermediate or intensive care monitoring. At a minimum, transcutaneous pacing pads are usually placed on the patient. A temporary transvenous pacing wire may be placed in cases of higher concern that the patient may develop asystole. A junctional escape rhythm is considered more stable than a ventricular escape rhythm. That is, the patient is less likely to suddenly develop asystole than when there is a ventricular escape rhythm (a ventricular escape rhythm is considered an unreliable escape rhythm)—although nothing is ever 100% predictable. Unless a reversible cause of the complete heart block is identified and can be easily treated (such as digoxin overdose), the patient is expeditiously treated with permanent pacemaker implantation.

Heartman's Clinical Pearl

It is sometimes confusing to those learning arrhythmia diagnosis whether an arrhythmia is due to complete heart block or to some type of tachyarrhythmia. The key in determining this is to compare the rate of the P waves with the rate of the QRS complexes. In complete heart block, we always see P waves occurring at a rate faster than the QRS complexes on the rhythm strip that result from either the junctional escape rhythm or the ventricular escape rhythm. Put more simply, we see more P waves than QRS complexes. These P waves have no fixed relationship to the QRS complexes since impulses from the SA node and atria are not conducted down the AV node. In contrast, in a tachyarrhythmia in which there is abnormal spontaneous depolarization of the AV node (resulting in a junctional tachycardia), a reentrant rhythm such as AVNRT or AVRT, or abnormal spontaneous depolarization of the ventricle (resulting in ventricular tachycardia), the P wave rate will either be slower than, or similar to, the QRS complex rate. In other words, there will be either more QRS complexes than P waves (such as can occur with ventricular tachycardia and P wave dissociation) or a similar number of P waves and QRS complexes (which may occur with junctional tachycardia, AVNRT, or AVRT).

CHAPTER 12

Diagnosing Bradyarrhythmias

Now that we have discussed the causes of bradyarrhythmias, we can set about discussing how to diagnose the cause of a bradyarrhythmia. We can break down the causes of a bradycardia into three basic rhythms:

1. Sinus bradycardia
2. Junctional rhythm
3. Heart block (either second-degree or complete heart block)

Similar to how we set about diagnosing the cause of a tachyarrhythmia, the key step in determining the rhythm in patients with bradycardia is looking for P waves, as we discuss below. We can again break down diagnosing any arrhythmia, in this case bradyarrhythmias, into using 3 basic questions:

1. Are there P waves a normal distance before each QRS complex?
   → *If so, the rhythm is sinus bradycardia.*
2. Are there no P waves a normal distance before each QRS complex?
   → *If so, the rhythm will likely be junctional rhythm.*
3. Are there more P waves than QRS complexes?
   → *If so, the rhythm is either second-degree or complete heart block.*

Sinus Bradycardia

If normal appearing P waves are seen occurring a normal distance before each QRS complex, the rhythm is sinus bradycardia, as shown in Figure 12.1.

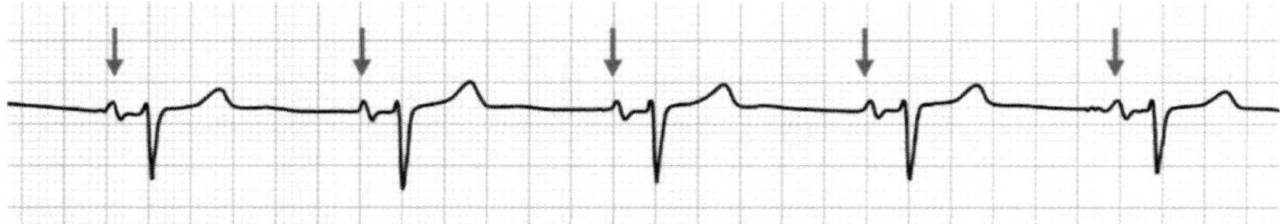

FIGURE 12.1. Sinus bradycardia. A P wave is seen before each QRS complex.

Junctional Rhythm

If no P waves are seen before each QRS complex and the QRS complexes are narrow and regular, then the rhythm is a junctional rhythm (Figure 12.2). Remember that junctional rhythms usually occur at a rate of 40–60 beats/min.

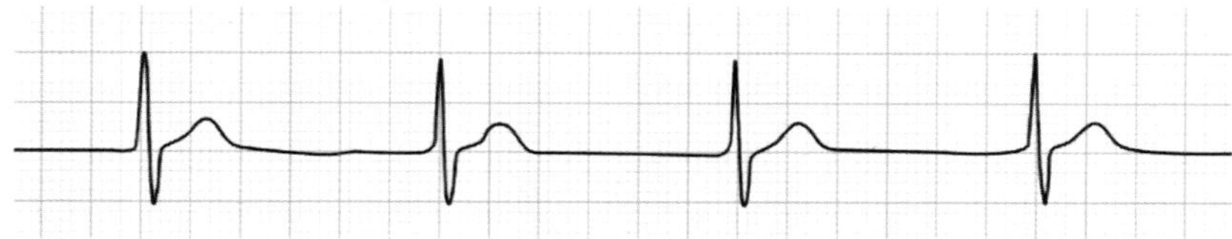

FIGURE 12.2. Junctional rhythm. No P waves are present before each QRS complex and the QRS complexes are narrow and regular, occurring at a rate of 50 beats/min.

Remember that occasionally in junctional rhythm, we see inverted P waves immediately before the QRS complexes, as the depolarization impulse generated by the AV node can sometime travel up into the atria and depolarize the atria in a bottom-to-top manner. Thus, the presence of inverted P waves *immediately before* the QRS complexes should not be mistaken for sinus rhythm or sinus bradycardia.

Second-Degree or Complete Heart Block

If there are more P waves than QRS complexes, then this is some type of second-degree or complete heart block. If some P waves are followed by a QRS complex, but some other P waves are not followed by a QRS complex, then the rhythm is second-degree heart block. Remember that there are two types of second-degree heart block (Mobitz type I, Wenkebach, and the more concerning Mobitz type II). If the PR interval progressively increases before the non-conducted P wave, then the rhythm is Mobitz type I second-degree heart block (Wenkebach), as shown in Figures 12.3 and 12.4.

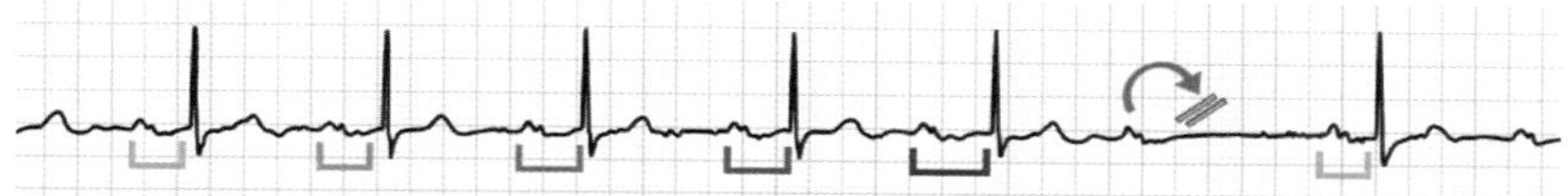

FIGURE 12.3. Mobitz type I second-degree heart block (Wenkebach). The PR interval progressively increases until there is a non-conducted P wave.

If instead there are constant PR intervals and then a non-conducted P wave suddenly occurs, the rhythm is Mobitz type II second-degree heart block (Figure 12.4).

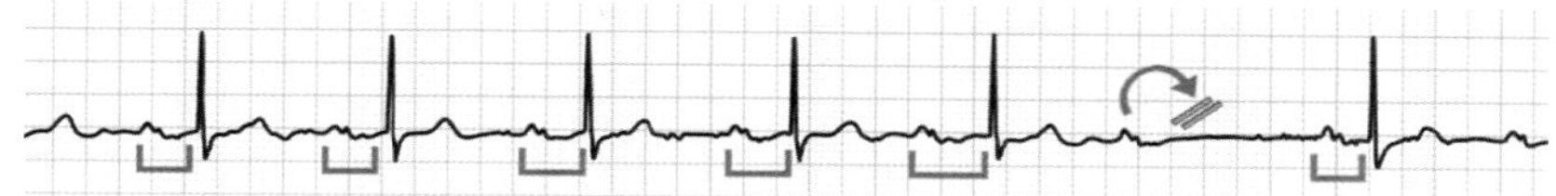

FIGURE 12.4. Mobitz type II second-degree heart block. The PR interval is constant until there an out of the blue non-conducted P wave appears.

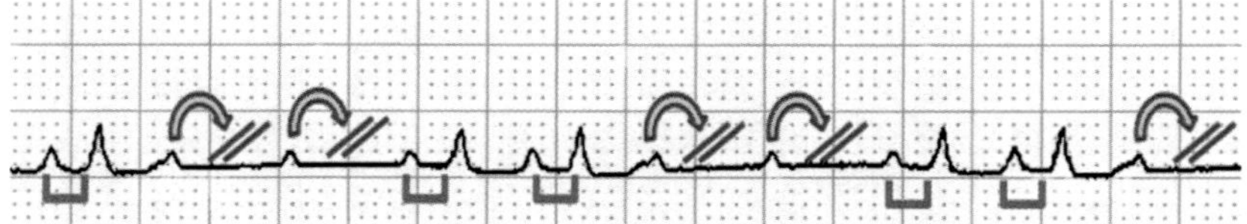

FIGURE 12.5. Another example of Mobitz type II second-degree heart block. There are periods where multiple P waves are not conducted until one finally gets through to the ventricle. This is "high-degree AV block" that is close to degenerating into complete heart block. This person urgently needs a pacemaker.

If P waves are present, occur at a rate faster than the QRS complexes, and are marching through the QRS complexes (have no fixed relationship to the QRS complexes), then the rhythm is third-degree (complete) heart block. If narrow complex QRS complexes are present at a regular rate, usually a rate of 40–60 beats/min, then the rhythm is complete heart block with a junctional escape rhythm (Figure 12.6).

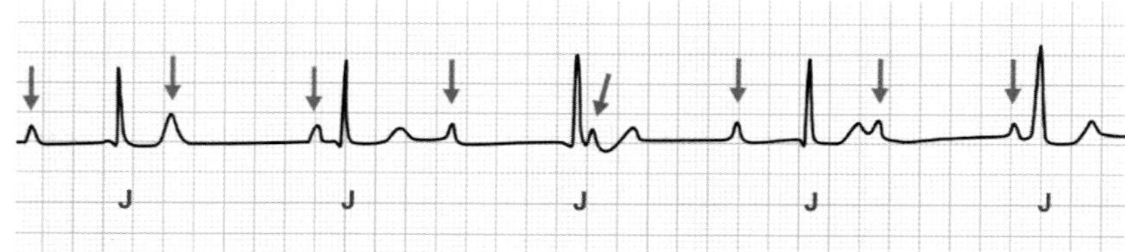

FIGURE 12.6. Third-degree (complete) heart block with a junctional escape rhythm. The P waves appear to march through the QRS complexes. Narrow QRS complexes (J for junctional escape beats) are present at a rate of about 40 beats/min.

If wide QRS complexes are present, usually at a rate of 30–40 beats/min, the rhythm is complete heart block with a ventricular escape rhythm (Figures 12.7 and 12.8).

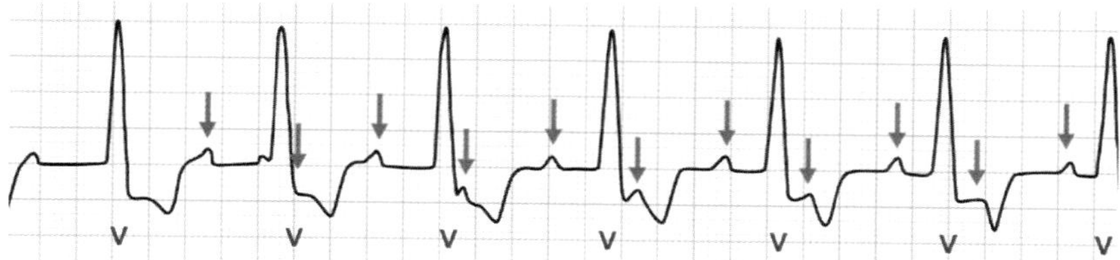

FIGURE 12.7. Third-degree (complete) heart block with a ventricular escape rhythm. The P waves appear to march through the QRS complexes. Wide QRS complexes are present due to the ventricular escape rhythm.

Heartman's Clinical Pearl

Occasionally, we come across a rhythm in which every other P wave is non-conducted. Because there is only one conducted P wave before there is a non-conducted P wave, we cannot tell if the PR interval is progressively increasing or not before there is a non-conducted P wave. Therefore, we cannot say whether this is Mobitz type I heart block (Wenkebach) or Mobitz type II heart block.

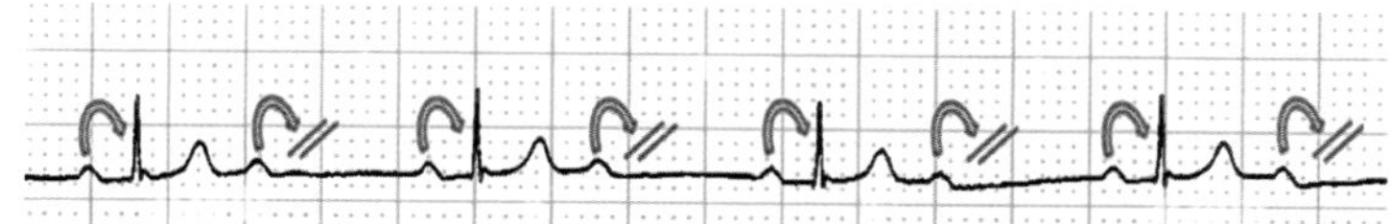

FIGURE 12.8. Second-degree heart block in which every other P wave is not conducted. This could be either Wenkebach or the more concerning Mobitz type II heart block.

Patients with acute inferior MI not infrequently develop second-degree heart block with this pattern of every other P wave being non-conducted. Inferior MI often leads to increased vagal tone, and in most such patients the cause of this heart block turns out to be Wenkebach, which is often caused by increased vagal stimulation of the AV node. In contrast, in patients with acute anterior MI, the arrhythmia is often due to Mobitz type II heart block, and suggests damage to the conduction system and the need for pacemaker placement. However, this is not a hard and fast rule, and either type of MI can lead to Mobitz type II heart block and ultimately complete heart block.

CHAPTER 13

Paced Rhythms

Paced rhythms often appear on first glance as arrhythmias—both bradyarrhythmias and tachyarrhythmias. Therefore, it is important to be familiar with paced rhythms and how to recognize them.

Pacemakers (Figure 13.1) are usually implanted if either the SA node is dysfunctional and the heart rate is too slow, or the AV node and conduction system becomes diseased and fails to normally conduct depolarization impulses from the SA node and atrium to the ventricles (Figure 13.2). In most patients, a pacemaker lead is placed in both the right atrium and in the right ventricle (Figure 13.2). These leads serve two functions:

- The leads allow the pacemaker to monitor the heart rhythm and determine if it needs to pace the atria and/or the ventricles.
- The leads also deliver electrical depolarization impulses to the atria and/or ventricles when needed—initiating depolarization of the atria and/or ventricles.

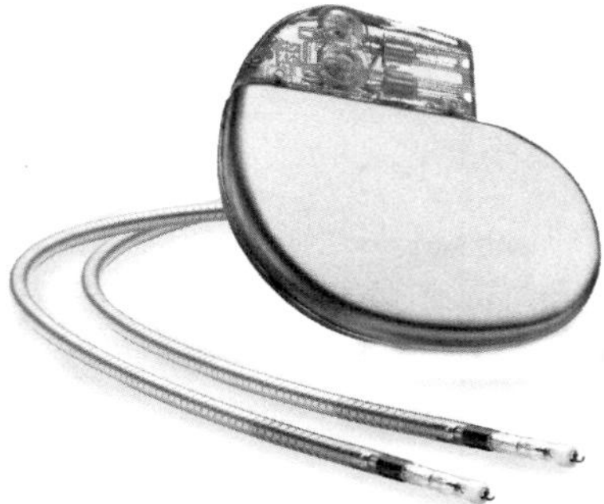

FIGURE 13.1. A typical pacemaker, with two leads.

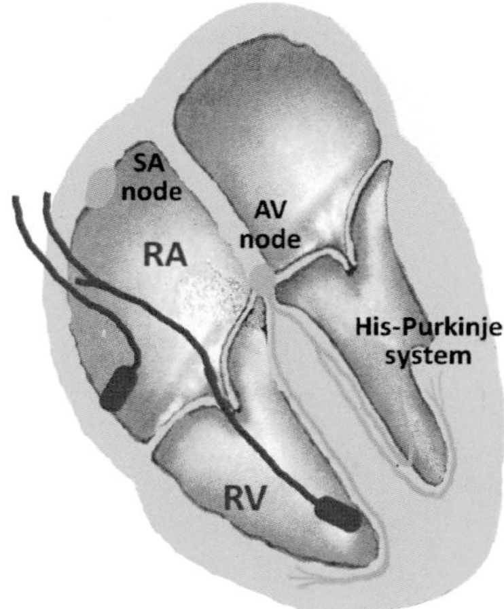

FIGURE 13.2. Pacemaker leads present in the right atrium (RA) and right ventricle (RV).

The way most modern pacemakers work is as follows. First, the pacemaker lead in the right atrium waits a programmed amount of time, waiting to see if it senses a depolarization impulse generated by the SA node. If it does, then the pacemaker realizes there is no need for it to generate a depolarization impulse itself. If it does *not* sense a native depolarization impulse and P wave, then the pacemaker goes ahead and generates a depolarization impulse. Whether the SA node generates a depolarization impulse or the pacemaker does this, the pacemaker then waits to see if the pacemaker lead in the right ventricle detects that the depolarization impulse has successfully made it down the AV node and His-Purkinje system into the ventricles. If it does detect that the depolarization impulse has made it to the ventricles, then it does not itself generate a depolarization impulse. If it does *not* sense that the depolarization impulse has made it to the ventricle, then it generates a depolarization impulse itself.

When the pacemaker generates a depolarization impulse, it appears on the ECG as a small vertical spike. It is important to become familiar with recognizing such pacemaker spikes so that a rhythm is not mistakenly identified as a bradyarrhythmia or tachyarrhythmia. We see examples of these pacemaker spikes in the ECGs that follow.

In some persons, the primary problem is a dysfunctional SA node. The AV node continues to be able to conduct impulses into the ventricle. In such patients, the pacemaker paces the atria only. As shown in Figure 13.3, the ECG demonstrates an atrial pacing spike (arrow) a short distance before each QRS complex. P waves are present immediately after the pacing spike. This rhythm is termed an atrial paced rhythm. Notice that the P waves in atrial paced rhythms are generally smaller and harder to see than the normal P waves seen in sinus rhythm.

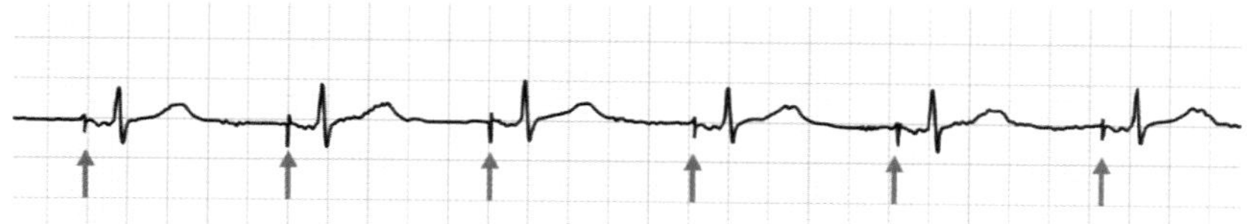

FIGURE 13.3. Atrial paced rhythm. Pacing spikes (arrows) and subtle P waves are present before each QRS complex (look carefully).

In other persons, the primary problem is an AV node and conduction system that cannot conduct depolarization impulses from the atria down into the ventricle. In these patients, the pacemaker senses that the SA node has generated a depolarization impulse but that depolarization impulse has not been conducted down in the ventricle. The pacemaker therefore paces the ventricle after each atrial depolarization. As shown in Figure 13.4, the ECG demonstrates a sinus tachycardia with pacer spikes immediately before each QRS complex. The pacemaker senses that there is a sinus tachycardia, and paces the ventricle at that rate. Note that paced QRS complexes are wide, since the His-Purkinje system is not involved in depolarizing the ventricle, and depolarization impulses generated by the pacemaker lead spread slowly across the ventricles. When the pacemaker correctly senses the P waves (atrial depolarization) and subsequently paces the ventricle, we say that there is "atrial sensing and ventricular pacing" present.

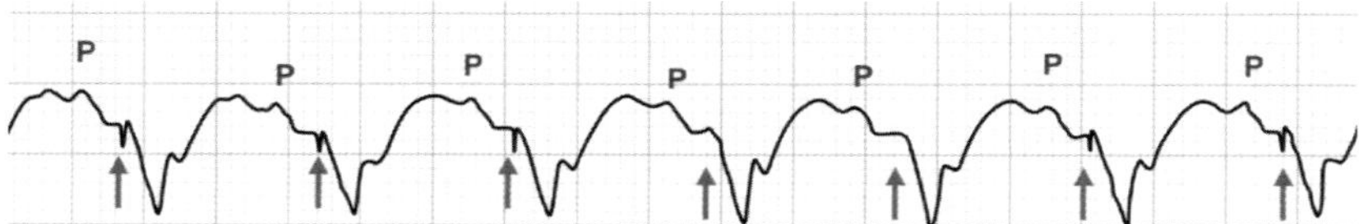

FIGURE 13.4. Ventricular paced rhythm. P waves (P) are followed by ventricular pacing spikes (arrows) and QRS complexes.

The tracing in Figure 13.5 is another example of a ventricular paced rhythm. Notice that if you did not recognize that there were ventricular pacing spikes present, you can easily mistake this rhythm as a wide complex tachycardia.

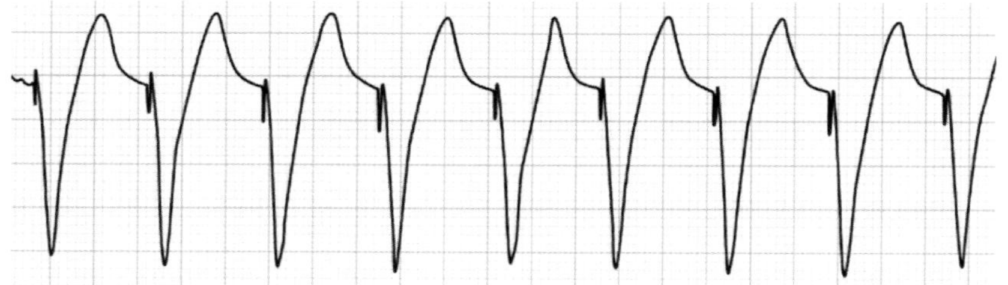

FIGURE 13.5. This ventricular paced rhythm could be mistaken for a wide complex tachycardia unless the pacer spikes immediately before the QRS complexes are noticed.

The ECG displayed in Figure 13.6 an example of AV sequential pacing. AV sequential pacing means that both the atria and ventricles are paced, with an atrial pacing impulse followed shortly thereafter by a ventricular pacing impulse. Both an atrial pacing spike and a ventricular pacing spike are present for each beat (note you must look carefully to see the ventricular pacing spikes, which is often the case!). The pacemaker is thus pacing both the atria and the ventricles, hence the name "AV sequential pacing".

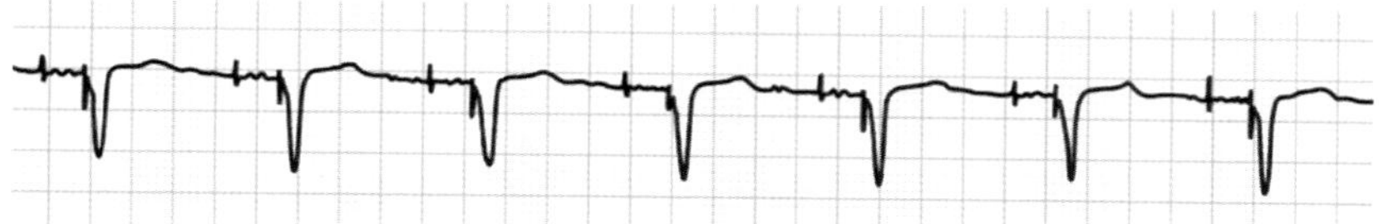

FIGURE 13.6. AV sequential pacing. There are both atrial and ventricular pacing spikes present.

Biventricular Pacing

These days, it is helpful to be aware of and understand a special type of ventricular pacing that is used to treat patients with heart function with reduced ejection fraction (HFrEF). This special type of pacing is referred to as "biventricular (biV) pacing" or "cardiac resynchronization therapy (CRT)".

The rationale for biV pacing is as follows. In some patients with heart failure due to reduced left ventricular ejection fraction (<40%), there is dyssynchronous contraction of the left ventricle's septal and lateral walls, leading to inefficient left ventricular contraction and pumping of blood into the body. This occurs where there is conduction system disease in the His-Purkinje system, often due to a left bundle branch block. BiV pacing has been found in patients with HFrEF and dyssynchronous ventricular contraction to improve symptoms, decrease hospitalizations for heart failure, and even decrease mortality. The benefit is most likely to be greatest in patients with a left bundle branch block and/or a QRS width of ≥150 msec.

In biV pacing, one pacer lead is, as usual, inserted into the right ventricle along the septal wall (usually near the apex). A second ventricular lead is inserted through the right atrium and coronary sinus, and then through the great cardiac vein and down a branch of this vein, so that the second pacer lead is adjacent to the lateral wall of the left ventricle (Figures 13.7–13.9). By adjusting the timing of when these two ventricular leads deliver a depolarization impulse to the septum and to the lateral wall of the left ventricle, more synchronized contraction of these walls and the entire left ventricle can occur, improving contractility and leading to long-term benefits.

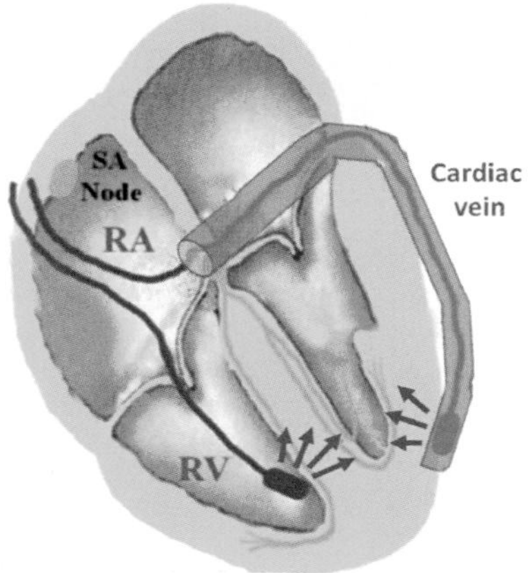

FIGURE 13.7. Biventricular pacing. In biV pacing, or CRT, one ventricular pacer lead is implanted, as usual, in the right ventricle, along the septum at the apex of the right ventricle. A second ventricular pacer lead is inserted into the right atrium, then through the coronary sinus and cardiac vein, adjacent to the lateral wall of the left ventricle. One lead thus depolarizes the left ventricle from the septal side (red arrows), while the other depolarizes the left ventricle from the lateral wall side (red arrows), leading to more synchronous contraction of the left ventricle.

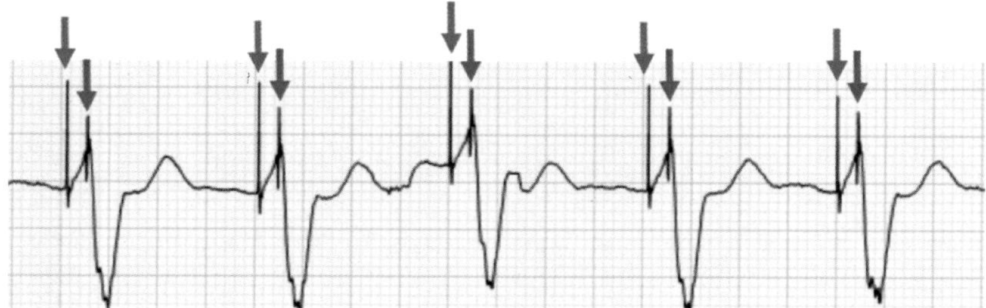

FIGURE 13.8. An example of the ECG tracing seen in biventricular pacing. Note the two distinct pacer spikes (red and blue arrows) before each QRS complex.

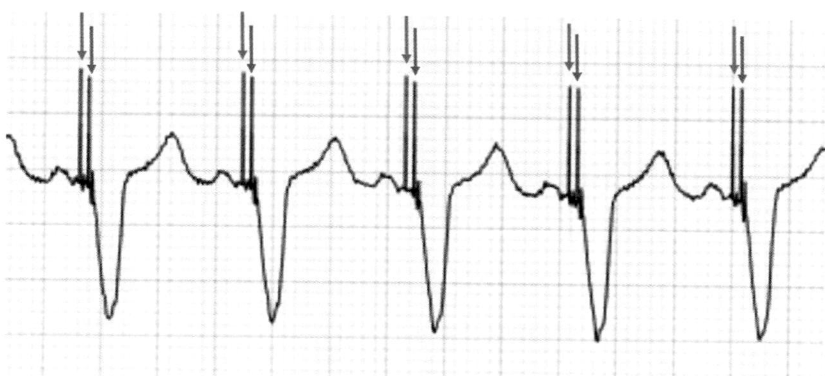

FIGURE 13.9. A second example of biventricular pacing, with two distinct pacer spikes (red and blue arrows) before each QRS complex. Sometimes these pacer spikes can be very close together and hard to distinguish.

Heartman's Clinical Pearl

Complicating things a little more, there is now another approach being used for ventricular pacing. This approach is to place the ventricular lead into the interventricular septum, high enough up that it can lead to synchronous pacing of the left bundle branch and right bundle branch. Placement of just the standard right ventricular pacing lead, near the apex, causes dyssynchronous ventricular depolarization and dyssynchronous ventricular contraction, which over time can lead to worsening ventricular function. Thus in some patients who require a pacemaker, this newer method of placing the ventricular lead high up in the septum is being used to avoid that potential complication. You may hear this type of pacing referred to as "septal pacing" or "His bundle pacing". This approach is also being used in patients with already depressed left ventricular function who already have dyssynchronous ventricular contraction, as an alternative to biventricular pacing.Patients with acute inferior MI not infrequently develop second-degree heart block with this pattern of every other P wave being non-conducted. Inferior MI often leads to increased vagal tone, and in most such patients the cause of this heart block turns out to be Wenkebach, which is often caused by increased vagal stimulation of the AV node. In contrast, in patients with acute anterior MI, the arrhythmia is often due to Mobitz type II heart block, and suggests damage to the conduction system and the need for pacemaker placement. However, this is not a hard and fast rule, and either type of MI can lead to Mobitz type II heart block and ultimately complete heart block.

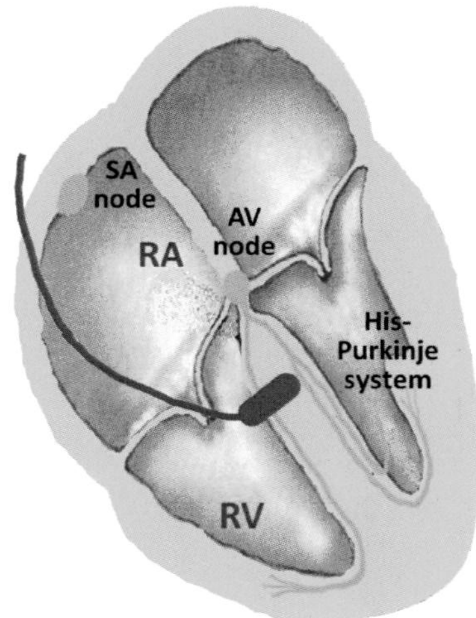

FIGURE 13.10. A newer form of pacing, called "septal pacing" or "His bundle pacing", in which the ventricular lead is inserted into the ventricular septum, high enough up in the conduction system to avoid or to treat dyssynchronous depolarization.

The resulting ECG strip shows a single ventricular pacing spike with a narrow QRS complex (Figure 13.11)

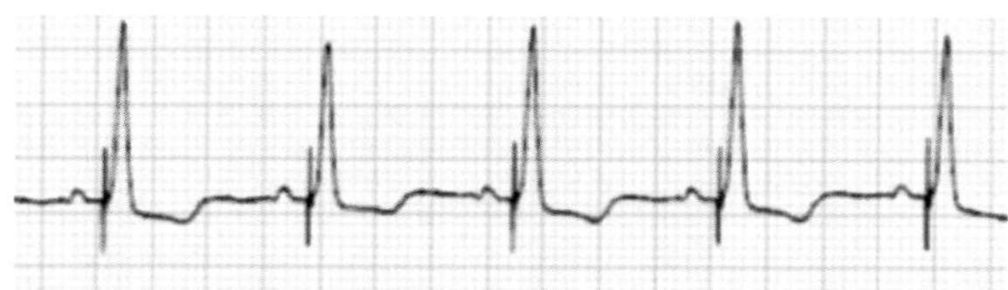

FIGURE 13.11. The ECG in His bundle pacing. A single ventricular pacing spike is followed by a narrow QRS complex.

CHAPTER 14

Miscellaneous Arrhythmias

Now that we have covered the basics of arrhythmias, we will briefly discuss a few other arrhythmias and ECG tracings that you will likely encounter while taking care of patients, and thus should be able to recognize.

The ECG shown in Figure 14.1 is an example of what is called "tachy-brady syndrome". The ECG shows that the patient initially has a fast heart rate due to atrial fibrillation. Midway through the ECG strip the atrial fibrillation terminates. There is a several-second pause until normal sinus rhythm resumes. Tachy-brady syndrome is an occasional cause of syncope, particularly in older patients. Such patients have paroxysmal atrial fibrillation (atrial fibrillation that spontaneously begins and terminates on its own). When the atrial fibrillation terminates, there is a several-second pause before normal sinus rhythm resumes. If this pause is more than three or four seconds, the patient may experience lightheadedness or even overt syncope. This condition is often referred to as "sick sinus syndrome", although "tachy-brady syndrome" is a better and more precise way to describe the arrhythmia and condition. Patients with tachy-brady syndrome often require placement of a permanent pacemaker.

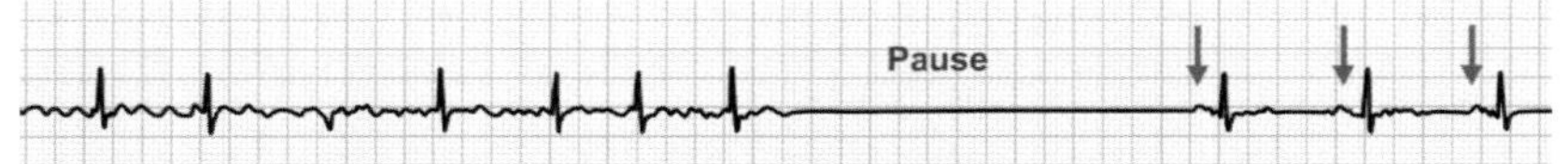

FIGURE 14.1. An example of tachy-brady syndrome (sick sinus syndrome). When the atrial fibrillation terminates, there is a several-second pause before normal sinus rhythm resumes.

The next rhythm is an example of atrial tachycardia with high-degree AV block, which is an arrhythmia that can occur with digoxin toxicity (Figure 14.2). There are unusual P waves occurring at a rate of 180 beats/min. Only one out of every four of these P waves appears to be conducted through the AV node, leading to ventricular depolarization and a QRS complex. Digoxin toxicity can "irritate" cells in the atria, leading to enhanced automaticity and spontaneous depolarization of this tissue, resulting in atrial tachycardia. At the same time, digoxin increases vagal tone on the AV node, which slows and decreases conduction down the AV node. The very high digoxin level leads to marked increased vagal tone on the AV node, and is a reason why there is only 4:1 conduction through the AV node (for every four atrial impulses, only one is conducted through the AV node down in to the ventricle). When we see atrial tachycardia with such high-degree AV block, think digoxin toxicity!

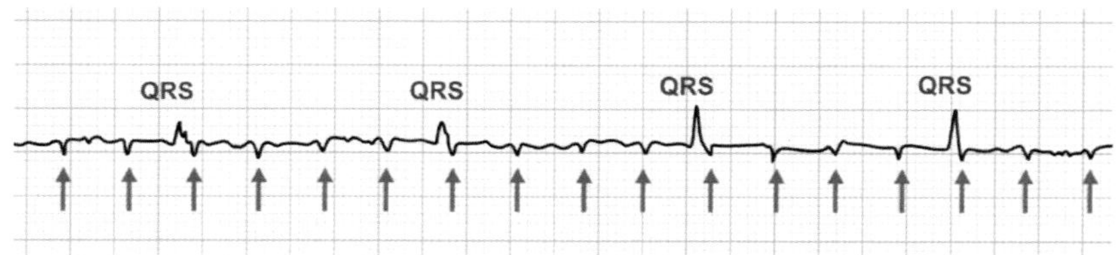

FIGURE 14.2. Atrial tachycardia with high-degree AV block, suggestive of digoxin toxicity. Only one out of every four P waves (arrows) is conducted.

Occasionally we see a rhythm where there is a normal P wave and QRS complex followed by a premature ventricular contraction (PVC), and this pattern repeats itself again and again. Such a rhythm is termed "ventricular bigeminy". If there are two normal

P waves and QRS complexes followed by a PVC in a repetitive pattern, the rhythm is called "ventricular trigeminy". If instead of a normal beat followed by a PVC, the normal beat is followed by an atrial premature contraction (APC) in a repetitive pattern, that rhythm is denoted as "atrial bigeminy". The ECG strip in Figure 14.3 shows an example of ventricular bigeminy.

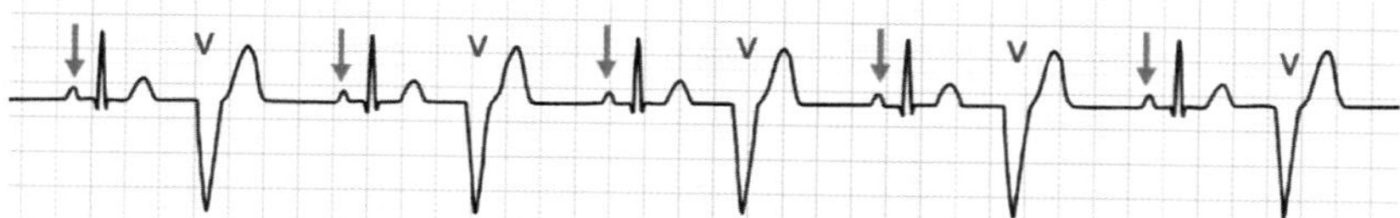

FIGURE 14.3. Ventricular bigeminy. Each normal P wave (red arrow) and QRS complex is followed by a premature ventricular contraction (V).

The next rhythm strips (Figure 14.4) show two examples of ventricular flutter. Ventricular flutter is an unstable ventricular arrhythmia that can be thought of as existing in a spectrum of ventricular arrhythmias between ventricular tachycardia and ventricular fibrillation. Ventricular flutter is an unstable arrhythmia that occurs at a rate of between 200 and 300 beats/min. There is little organized ventricular contraction in ventricular flutter, and thus patients are often pulseless and unresponsive. The rhythm often quickly degenerates to ventricular fibrillation. Treatment of patients with ventricular flutter is immediate defibrillation.

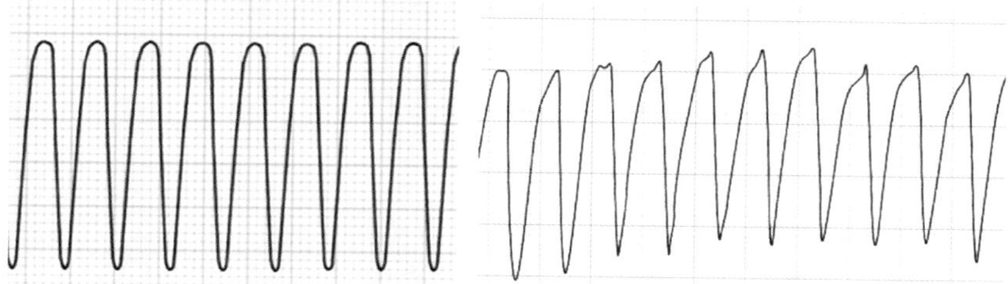

FIGURE 14.4. Two examples of ventricular flutter.

The rhythm strip in Figure 14.5 is an example of an unusual ECG tracing that we mentioned before in a previous chapter. This rhythm strip shows the ECG tracing that occurs when someone who has a bypass tract (such as in Wolff-Parkinson-White syndrome) develops atrial fibrillation. The rhythm is irregular and the QRS complexes are of varying width. The QRS impulses are of varying width because some of the impulses that reach and depolarize the ventricle travel down the AV node and His-Purkinje system, resulting in narrow QRS complexes, while some other impulses that depolarize the ventricle travel down the bypass tract, resulting in wide QRS complexes. Further, sometimes impulses traveling down the AV node and His-Purkinje system and impulses traveling down the bypass tract arrive in the ventricle at the same time, resulting in QRS complexes that are a hybrid of a narrow QRS complex and a wide QRS complex. The resulting rhythm strip is essentially a montage of narrow QRS complexes, wide QRS complexes, and QRS complexes of intermediate width. As previously discussed, patients who develop this arrhythmia should not be treated with medications that slow conduction down the AV node (including amiodarone), as this may somewhat paradoxically lead to an increase in heart rate as more impulses travel down the bypass tract and depolarize the ventricles, and can lead the patient to develop ventricular fibrillation.

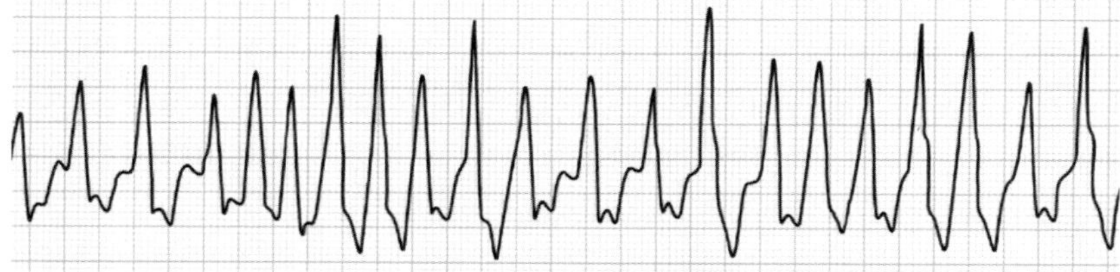

FIGURE 14.5. The ECG tracing that results when someone with a bypass tract develops atrial fibrillation. There is marked variation in the QRS complex morphologies and RR intervals.

Look at this unusual ECG tracing in Figure 14.6. Not uncommonly, this will occur and the telemetry alarm goes off. While at first this appears to be some bizarre arrhythmia, on careful inspection one can see that there are normal appearing QRS complexes (arrows), distinct from everything else on the ECG tracing. This is an example of artifact, and how artifact can initially appear to be an arrhythmia. Common causes of artifact include shivering, seizure, tremor, and even toothbrushing.

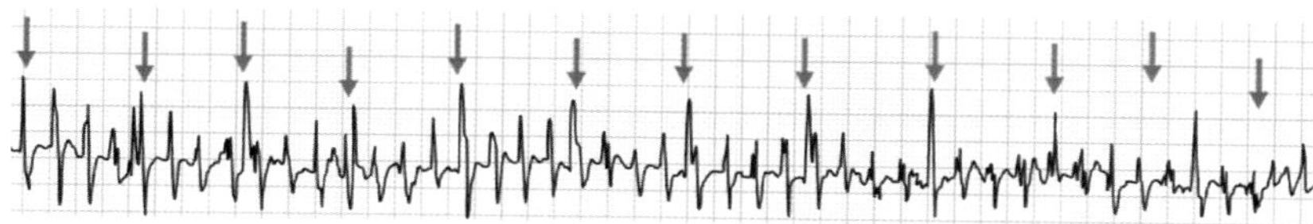

FIGURE 14.6. An example of an ECG tracing with artifact. Notice the larger QRS complexes (arrows) occurring at regular intervals. The smaller deflections occurring at a very fast rate are artifact.

The ECG tracing in Figure 14.7 is another example of artifact. There are several important keys to recognizing that this is artifact. First, in the mid-portion of the ECG strip, there are the bizarre narrow deflections occurring at a very fast rate. Such deflections are not easily explained by any real arrhythmia. Second, the "arrhythmia" seems to start while we can still see normal QRS complexes. Third, immediately upon termination of this "arrhythmia," we see normal QRS complexes occurring. In most cases of tachyarrhythmias, when the arrhythmia breaks there is usually a short pause before normal sinus rhythm resumes. It would be highly unusual to see normal QRS complexes from normal sinus rhythm occurring essentially immediately as the arrhythmia terminates.

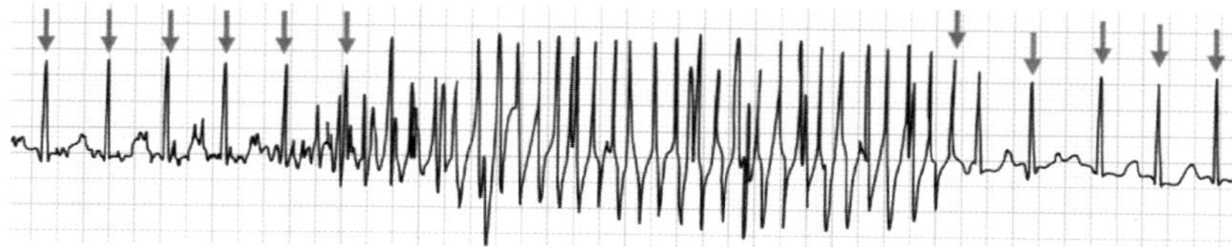

FIGURE 14.7. Another example of artifact. The "arrhythmia" seems to start while there are still normal QRS complexes, and normal QRS complexes are again seen immediately as the "arrhythmia" terminates. These are important clues that this is artifact instead of an actual arrhythmia.

CHAPTER 15

BLS and ACLS Treatment of Arrhythmias

Basic life support (BLS) and advanced cardiac life support (ACLS) are best learned through a dedicated course, such as those designed by the American Heart Association (AHA). In this chapter, we will briefly review some of the most important aspects of BLS and ACLS as it relates to the treatment of three basic types of arrhythmias:

1. Ventricular fibrillation (VF) and pulseless ventricular tachycardia (VT)
2. Tachycardia with a pulse
3. Bradyarrhythmias

Ventricular Fibrillation and Pulseless Ventricular Tachycardia

The simplified BLS algorithm for health-care providers emphasizes the following steps:

1. Assess if the patient is unresponsive and not breathing (or only abnormally gasping for breathes).
2. Activate the emergency medical response system and get an automated external defibrillator (AED) or manual cardioverter/defibrillator.
3. Check for a pulse. Spend no more than ten seconds doing this.
4. Begin CPR (cycles of thirty chest compressions and two breaths, beginning with thirty chest compressions).

5. Check for a shockable rhythm as soon as the AED/defibrillator arrives. Shockable rhythms in such settings are VF and VT. Give one shock ASAP.

The simplified BLS algorithm is shown in the Figure 15.1. It emphasizes cycles of good quality CPR and defibrillation (if indicated) as soon as possible.

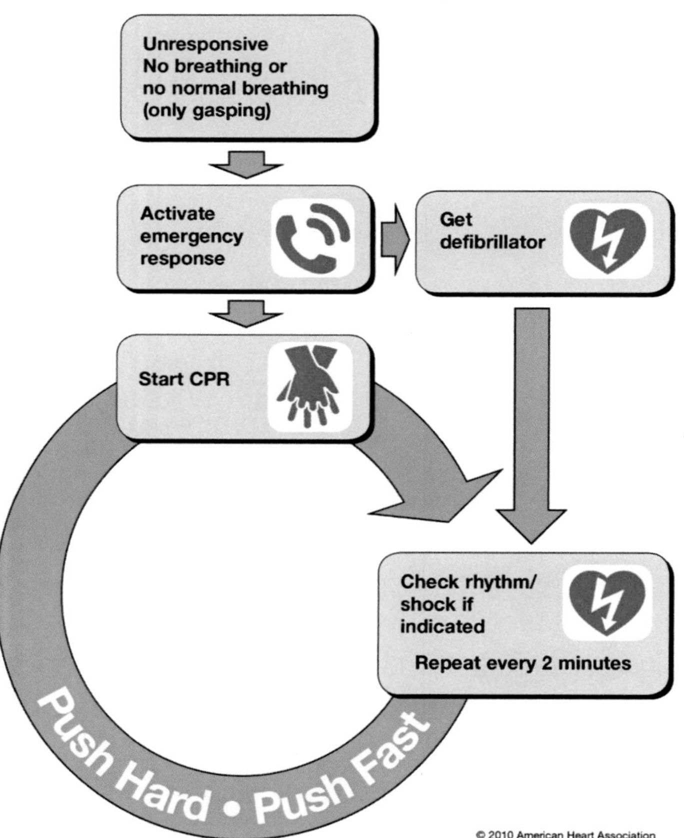

FIGURE 15.1. The simplified adult BLS algorithm. Reproduced with permission from 2010 American Heart Association Guidelines Update for CPR and ECC – Part 5: Adult Basic Life Support. Circulation. 2010;122:S685–S705.). ©2010, American Heart Association, Inc.

Heartman's Clinical Pearl

Irreversible brain damage begins to occur as early as four minutes after the brain is deprived of oxygen, such as occurs during pulseless cardiac arrest. In patients who develop witnessed VF and cardiac arrest, survival rates decrease 7%–10% for every minute that passes until successful defibrillation if no bystander CPR is provided. Even with bystander CPR, survival rates fall 3%–4% per minute until successful defibrillation. In patients who are not successfully defibrillated within minutes of cardiac arrest, survival with intact cognitive function is dismal. Survival rates with "code blue" are much higher in patients with VF or pulseless VT who are quickly defibrillated than is survival with other rhythms (such as pulseless electrical activity [PEA] or asystole). Therefore, the single key driving force when treating the patient with arrhythmia and cardiac arrest, is to as quickly as possible determine if the patient is in VF or pulseless VT and immediately defibrillate the patient.

The ACLS algorithm for VF and pulseless VT (VT without a pulse) involves the same basic concept as the BLS algorithm of prompt defibrillation and two-minute cycles of CPR. It additionally incorporates obtaining IV or intraosseous (IO) access to administer drugs, the administration of certain drugs, and use of an advanced airway (eg, intubation). The initial steps in the ACLS algorithm for VF and pulseless VT include recognizing that the patient is non-responsive, activating the emergency medical response system, obtaining an AED or manual cardioverter/defibrillator, and starting CPR. The patient should be defibrillated as soon as an AED/defibrillator is available if the rhythm is determined to be VF or pulseless VT.

In newer ACLS guidelines, as soon as the first shock is delivered, CPR should immediately be resumed and continued for two minutes before the rhythm is reassessed or a pulse check is performed. When IV or IO access is established, the vasopressor drug (one that constricts the blood vessels) epinephrine (1 mg) should be administered. After two minutes of CPR since the first shock, the rhythm and pulse are reassessed. If the patient remains in VF or VT, then another shock is delivered. CPR is again immediately resumed for two more minutes. If the patient remains in VF or VT, the antiarrhythmic drug amiodarone can be administered (the first dose is a 300 mg bolus).

A simplified version of the ACLS algorithm is shown in Figure 15.2. Key points emphasized in the new ACLS guidelines include the following:

- CPR should be initiated as soon as possible. The regimen is thirty compressions and two breaths.
- Defibrillation should be performed as soon as possible.
- Immediately after a shock is delivered, CPR is resumed for two minutes before the rhythm is reassessed and a pulse check is performed.
- Epinephrine can be administered when IV (or IO) access is established.
- If the patient remains in VF or VT despite multiple shocks, the antiarrhythmic agent amiodarone can be administered.

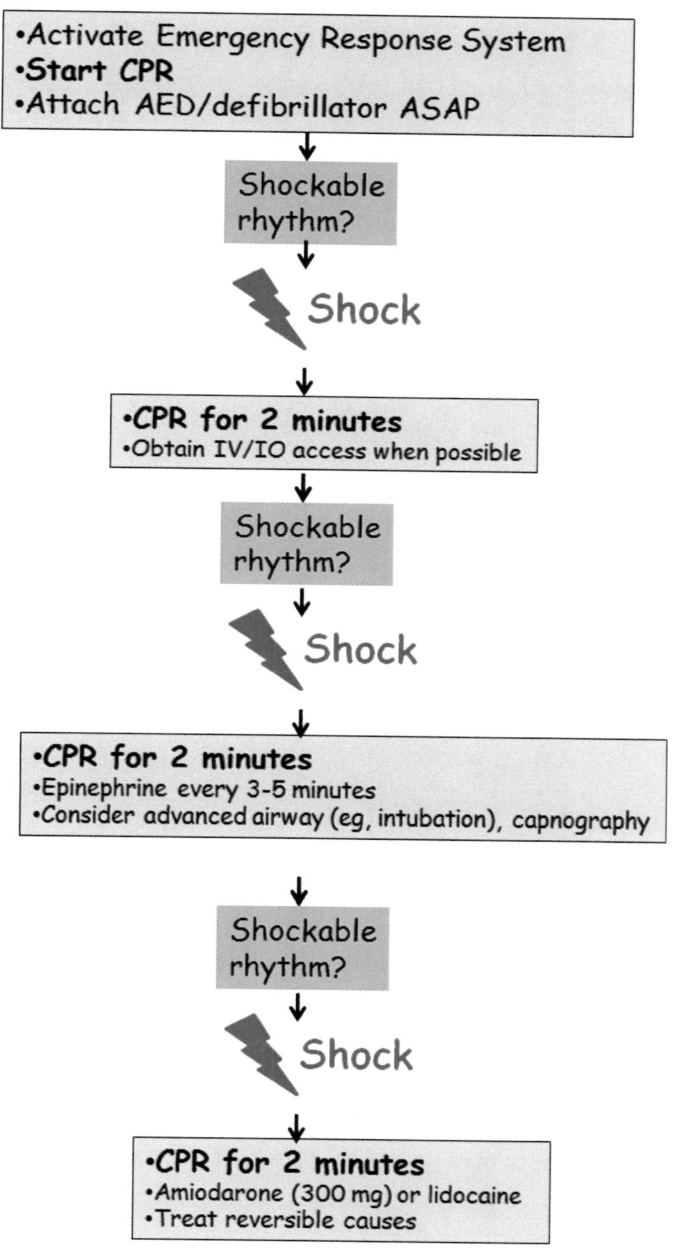

FIGURE 15.2. A simplified ACLS algorithm for VF and pulseless VT. Adopted from American Heart Association 2020 Advanced Cardiac Life Support Provider Manual – Adult Cardiac Arrest Algorithm. American Heart Association, Inc.

Heartman's Clinical Pearl

The energy level used for defibrillation of VF or pulseless VT depends on whether the defibrillator delivers a monophasic or biphasic shock, as well as the manufacturer of the defibrillator. The energy level for AEDs is pre-set, so when using an AED deciding what energy to choose is not an issue. When using a manual cardioverter/defibrillator that delivers a biphasic shock, which most recently manufactured devices are, the recommended energy level is usually 120–200 joules (J), depending upon the manufacturer of the device. If the recommended energy level for defibrillation is not known, the ACLS protocol suggests using the maximum energy level of the device. For devices that deliver a monophasic shock, which are primarily older devices, an energy level of 360 J is recommended.

Tachycardia with a Pulse

Below are key highlights from the 2020 ACLS algorithm for tachycardia with a pulse (ACLS guidelines are updated every few years, so it is always advisable to review the latest iteration of this and all algorithms). ACLS guidelines for tachycardia with a pulse emphasize several important factors to be considered in the treatment of tachyarrhythmias:

- Assess whether the patient is asymptomatic or is symptomatic and unstable.
- Serious symptoms and signs that would classify the rhythm as an "unstable tachycardia" and warrant urgent treatment include hypotension, acutely altered mental status, signs of shock, ischemic chest discomfort, and acute heart failure.
- It is important to try to determine whether the tachycardia is a cause of the symptom or a result of the symptom and underlying medical condition.
- Ventricular heart rates <150 beats/min usually do not cause serious signs or symptoms (unless the patient has a severely reduced left ventricular ejection fraction or severe coronary artery disease).

- The approach to the arrhythmia may vary depending on whether it is a narrow complex tachycardia or a wide complex tachycardia.

The ACLS tachycardia with a pulse algorithm is one algorithm that addresses both narrow and wide complex tachycardias. For the purposes of simplicity, however, the algorithm here is divided into two separate algorithms, one for narrow complex tachycardias with a pulse (Figure 15.3) and one for wide complex tachycardias with a pulse (Figure 15.5). This is consistent with our general approach in diagnosing arrhythmias to decide whether the QRS complexes are narrow or wide.

The initial step in the algorithm is to identify and treat any underlying cause of the arrhythmia and to take several steps to monitor and support the patient. The next step is to determine whether the tachycardia is causing severe symptoms. Treatment depends on whether the tachyarrhythmia is causing severe symptoms or not.

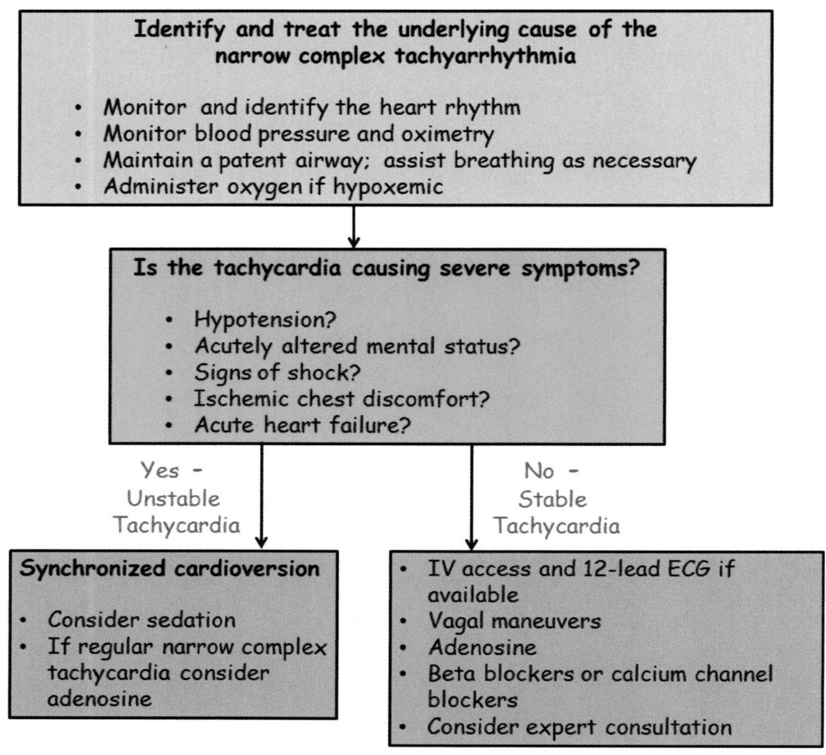

FIGURE 15.3. A simplified ACLS algorithm for the management of a patient with narrow complex tachycardia with a pulse. Adapted from the American Heart Association *Advanced Cardiac Life Support Provider Manual* – Adult Tachycardia with a Pulse Algorithm. American Heart Association, Inc.

Heartman's Clinical Pearl

In synchronized cardioversion, the cardioverter/defibrillator monitors the heart rhythm while shocking the heart, so that the shock is not inadvertently delivered to the heart during the vulnerable period (a period of repolarization during the cardiac cycle that corresponds to the T wave). A shock delivered to the heart during the vulnerable period while the heart is repolarizing can cause ventricular fibrillation. Cardioverter/defibrillators can deliver unsynchronized defibrillation shocks to the heart using the two "quick look" pads. However, to give synchronized shocks, be aware that some devices need additional leads to be connected to the patient, so that the device can monitor the heart rhythm using these leads and deliver the actual shock using the quick look pads. You usually need to push the "synchronize" button on the cardioverter/defibrillator to tell the device that you want to deliver a synchronized shock. If the cardioverter/defibrillator is ready to deliver a synchronized shock, small triangles, squares, circles, or arrows display on the device's monitor above each QRS complex, as shown in Figure 15.4. This demonstrates that the device is successfully recognizing and tracking the QRS complexes, the period in the cardiac cycle when the shock is delivered.

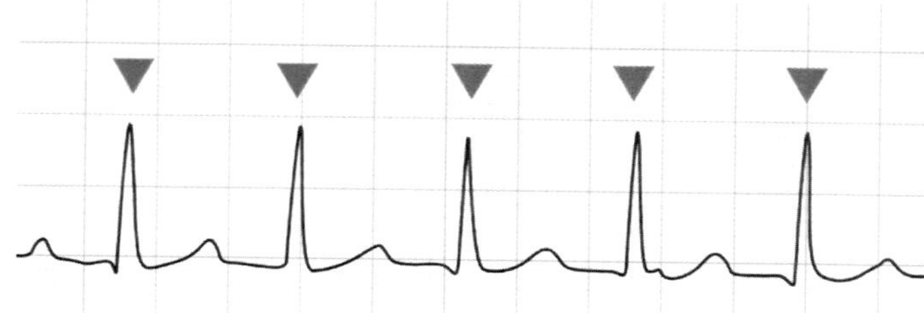

FIGURE 15.4. An example of the display on a cardioverter/defibrillator showing that the device is successfully tracking the QRS complexes. This particular device displays triangles above each QRS complex to demonstrate it can see and track the QRS complexes.

Adenosine is a quick- and short-acting drug that blocks conduction down the AV node. It is extremely effective for terminating AVNRT and AVRT, which as you remember are reentrant arrhythmias that involve the AV node. It may occasionally also terminate atrial tachycardia. The initial dose is 6 mg rapid IV push, followed by a normal saline flush of 20 cc. A second dose of 12 mg can be administered if the first dose fails to break the arrhythmia. Beta blockers and calcium channel blockers both slow conduction through the AV node. These drugs may therefore also terminate AVNRT or AVRT. They will slow the ventricular response rate if the arrhythmia is atrial fibrillation or atrial flutter, but not terminate such arrhythmias. Adenosine usually has little effect on the ventricular rate if the rhythm is atrial tachycardia or multifocal atrial tachycardia (MAT).

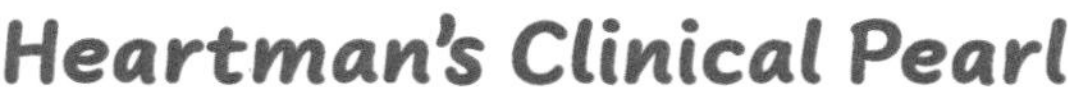

Heartman's Clinical Pearl

Remember that rhythms such as MAT and junctional tachycardia are due to enhanced automaticity of cells and not due to a reentrant arrhythmia. Because of this, cardioversion usually does not terminate these arrhythmias when they occur. Most cases of atrial tachycardia are also due to enhanced automaticity, and similarly will not be terminated by cardioversion.

The approach to a wide complex tachycardia is similar to that of a narrow complex tachycardia with a couple exceptions. Adenosine should only be considered if the patient is stable and the QRS complexes are regular and monomorphic. Adenosine might terminate the rhythm if it is a SVT (such as AVNRT or AVRT) with BBB. Antiarrhythmic treatment with agents such as procainamide or amiodarone can be considered to terminate the arrhythmia. Procainamide is infused at a rate of 20–50 mg/min until the arrhythmia terminates, hypotension ensues, the QRS width increases >50%, or a maximum dose of 17 mg/kg has been administered. Amiodarone is given as a first dose of 150 mg over ten minutes.

The approach to the patient with a wide complex tachycardia and a pulse is described in Figure 15.5.

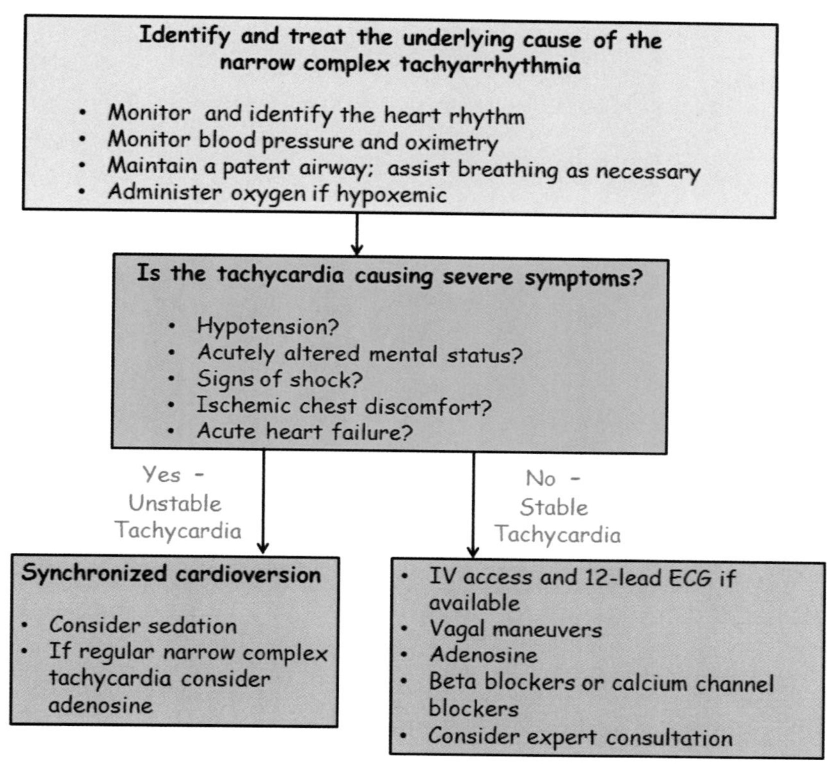

FIGURE 15.5. A simplified ACLS algorithm for the management of a patient with wide complex tachycardia with a pulse. Adapted from the American Heart Association 2020 *Advanced Cardiac Life Support Provider Manual* – Adult Tachycardia with a Pulse Algorithm. American Heart Association, Inc.

Bradycardia (with Pulse)

As we have discussed, there are many different arrhythmias that can cause bradycardia. The ACLS algorithm addresses the more general entity of bradycardia from any cause. Key aspects of the ACLS algorithm for bradycardia include:

- Identifying and treating the underlying cause.
- Assessing if the patient is symptomatic.
- Initial treatment with atropine.

- Treatment with either a medication that increases the heart rate (dopamine or epinephrine) or transcutaneous pacing if atropine treatment is ineffective.
- Expert consultation and/or transvenous pacing if necessary.

Symptoms that warrant acute treatment, if they are believed to be caused by the bradycardia and not some other medical condition, include hypotension, acutely altered mental status, signs of shock, ischemic chest discomfort, and acute heart failure. In such cases, the initial treatment is atropine. Atropine acts to decrease vagal stimulation of the heart, and thereby increases depolarization of the SA node and increases conduction down the AV node. The dose of atropine for symptomatic bradycardia is 1.0 mg IV (note that this an increased dose compared to older recommendations to give 0.5 mg). This dose is repeated every three to five minutes, up to a maximum total dose of 3 mg.

If atropine is ineffective, then the bradycardia is treated with either infusion of a drug that increases the heart rate or transcutaneous pacing. In unstable patients, particularly those with heart block, transcutaneous pacing is the first-line treatment if IV access cannot quickly be established to administer atropine. Drugs that can increase the heart rate that can be used in the setting of symptomatic bradycardia include dopamine and epinephrine. Dopamine infusion is typically at a rate of 5–20 mcg/kg/min and titrated to patient response. Epinephrine infusion is begun at a dose of 2–10 mcg/min and titrated to patient response.

The adult bradycardia with pulse algorithm is presented in Figure 15.6.

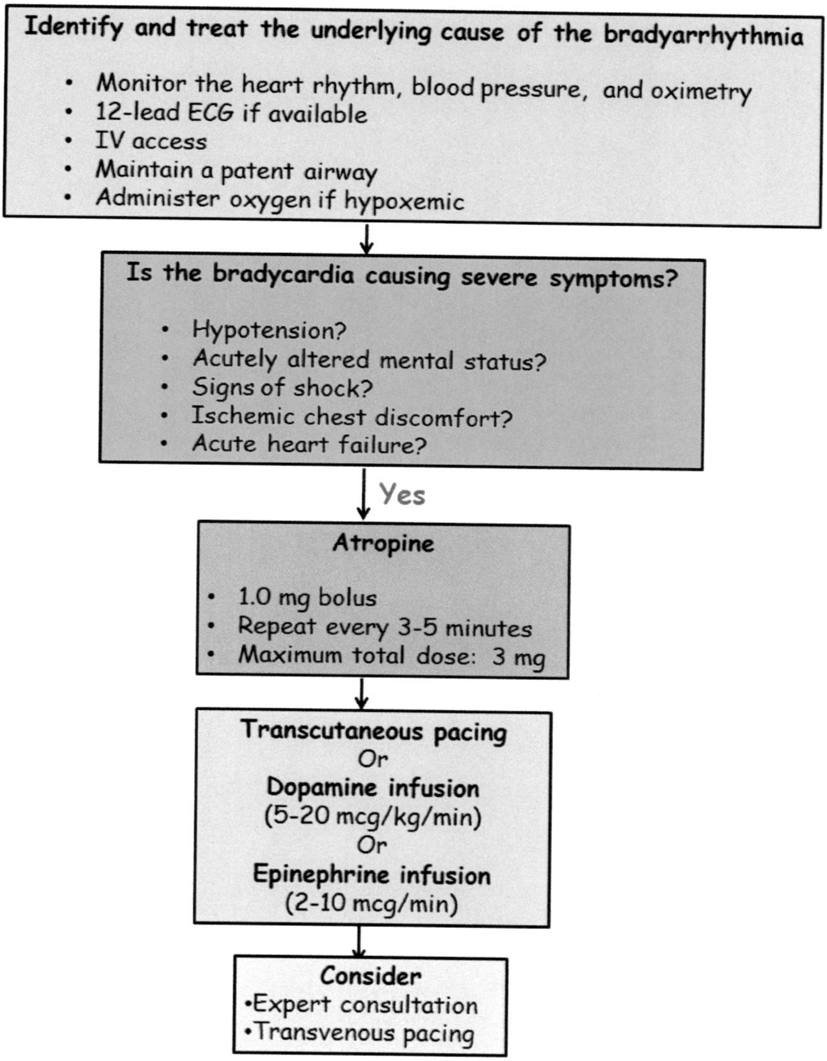

Identify and treat the underlying cause of the bradyarrhythmia

- Monitor the heart rhythm, blood pressure, and oximetry
- 12-lead ECG if available
- IV access
- Maintain a patent airway
- Administer oxygen if hypoxemic

↓

Is the bradycardia causing severe symptoms?

- Hypotension?
- Acutely altered mental status?
- Signs of shock?
- Ischemic chest discomfort?
- Acute heart failure?

↓ Yes

Atropine

- 1.0 mg bolus
- Repeat every 3-5 minutes
- Maximum total dose: 3 mg

↓

Transcutaneous pacing
Or
Dopamine infusion
(5-20 mcg/kg/min)
Or
Epinephrine infusion
(2-10 mcg/min)

↓

Consider
•Expert consultation
•Transvenous pacing

FIGURE 15.6. Simplified ACLS algorithm for adult bradycardia with pulse. Adapted with permission from the *Advanced Cardiac Life Support Provider Manual*.

CHAPTER 16

Summary

Most tachyarrhythmias can be easily diagnosed if we take a systematic approach to the arrhythmia. For tachycardias, we use this simple three-step approach of:

1. Determine if the QRS complexes seen in the arrhythmia are narrow or wide.
2. Determine if the QRS complexes occur at regular or irregular intervals.
3. Determine if there is any evidence of P waves or atrial activity present.

If the rhythm is a narrow complex regular tachycardia, there are only six possible causes: sinus tachycardia, atrial tachycardia, atrial flutter, junctional tachycardia, AVNRT, or AVRT. If the rhythm is a narrow complex irregular tachycardia, there are only three possible causes: multifocal atrial tachycardia (MAT), atrial flutter with variable conduction (variable block) down the AV node, and atrial fibrillation. Looking for P waves or atrial activity usually allows us to make the specific diagnosis of which arrhythmia is causing the narrow complex tachycardia.

For wide complex tachycardias, the rhythm in almost all cases is either SVT with BBB or VT. We use a slightly modified approach to determine the cause of the tachyarrhythmia:

1. Determine if the QRS complexes are narrow or wide (we've already decided that it is wide).
2. Determine if the QRS complexes are perfectly regular or slightly irregular.
3. Determine if P waves or evidence of atrial activity are present before each QRS complex, or if there is evidence of P wave (or AV) dissociation.

The presence of perfectly regular wide QRS complexes suggests the rhythm is an SVT, though we need to keep in mind that monomorphic VT can sometimes appear pretty regular. Slightly irregular QRS complexes favor a diagnosis of VT. Very irregular QRS complexes are usually due to polymorphic VT (though remember that atrial fibrillation in a patient with WPW can produce notable irregular QRS complexes). P waves or atrial activity before each QRS complex strongly suggests an SVT. P wave dissociation (AV dissociation) is almost always associated with VT.

Bradyarrhythmias may be due to one of three basic causes:

1. Sinus bradycardia
2. Junctional rhythm
3. Second-degree or third-degree (complete) heart block

Looking for P waves can allow us to make the diagnosis in most cases. If the P wave rate is faster than the QRS rate (or there are more P waves than QRS complexes), then heart block must be present.

When coming upon an arrhythmia, whether a bradyarrhythmia or tachyarrhythmia, we should always look carefully to see if pacer spikes are present. Sinus tachycardia with a paced ventricular rhythm can be easily mistaken for a wide complex tachycardia if we do not notice the small pacer spikes at the beginning of the QRS complexes.

ACLS algorithms emphasize the importance of activating an emergency medical response system, quickly obtaining an AED or manual cardioverter/defibrillator, initiating high quality CPR, and prompt cardioversion if the patient is unstable and immediate defibrillation if the patient is pulseless. Remember, brain death begins within minutes in the pulseless person with VF or VT, and immediate defibrillation is paramount.

We have finished your introductory course on arrhythmias. You should now have a basic understanding of what causes arrhythmias, where and how they occur in the heart, and how to diagnose and treat them. Heartman and I congratulate you on a job well done!

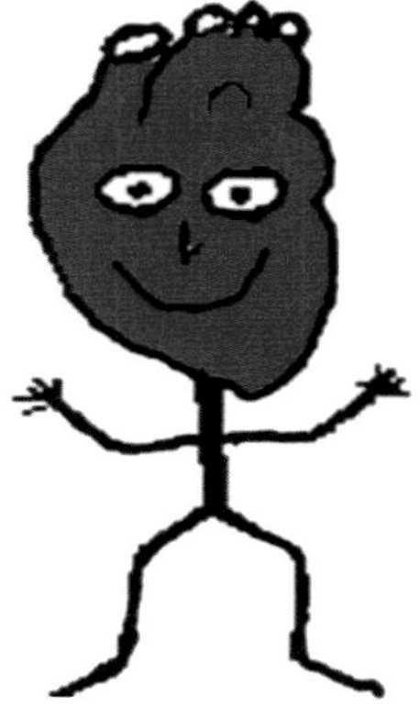

Acknowledgments

Special thanks to David Wogahn and his team at AuthorImprints for their wise counsel, cover design, and assistance with book formatting for publication.

About the Author

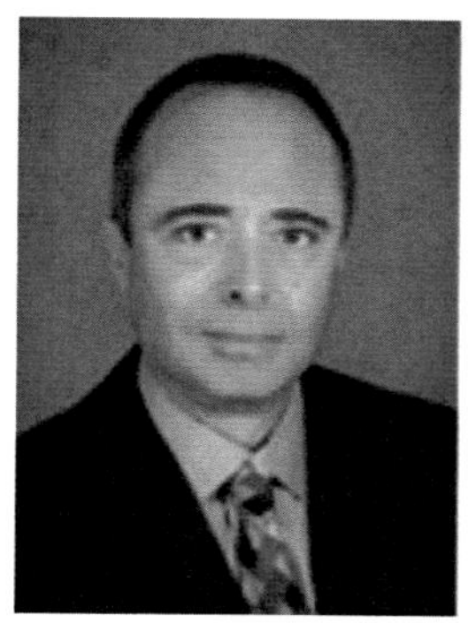

DR. GLENN N. LEVINE is Master Clinician and Professor of Medicine at Baylor College of Medicine, and Chief of Cardiology Section at the Michael E. DeBakey VA Medical Center, both in Houston Texas. Dr. Levine is recognized locally, regionally, nationally and internationally for his teaching, lecturing, and educational abilities, and for his expertise in cardiovascular disease.

Dr. Levine is the recipient of six Baylor College of Medicine Fulbright & Jaworski and Norton Rose Fulbright faculty excellence awards. He was awarded the prestigious Baylor College of Medicine Master Clinician Lifetime Award, recognizing his clinical skills and abilities to educate others on the management of patients with cardiovascular disease, as well as the Baylor College of Medicine's Presidential Award for Excellence in Education, the college's highest such honor. Dr. Levine's clinical and educational leadership have also been recognized by the American Heart Association, who awarded him their Council on Clinical Cardiology Distinguished Achievement Award, and by the American College of Cardiology, who awarded him the prestigious Gifted Educator Award, a national award bestowed upon only one cardiologist each year.

Dr. Levine has authored or edited a total of 16 educational textbooks and handbooks, including a 1000+ page textbook and atlas on cardiovascular disease. Several of these books have additionally been published internationally in different languages, including Russian, Lithuanian, Vietnamese, and Spanish. He has led and first-authored seven American Heart Association Scientific Statements. He has served as chair of multiple American College of Cardiology/American Heart Association guidelines and guideline focused updates. Recently, Dr. Levine served as chair of the American College of Cardiology/American Heart Association Task Force on Clinical Practice Guidelines, leading and supervising all of the nation's cardiovascular guidelines.

More recently, Dr. Levine's focuses have been on the more global relationship of the heart and mind, how psychological health affects the heart, and on the interrelated topics of meditation, mindfulness and well-being.

Socially, Dr. Levine is a passionate advocate of animal rescue and adoption, and the humane treatment of animals, belonging to over a dozen such advocate and animal rescue organizations (in addition to having numerous rescue dogs himself—all his life), and practices a balanced approach to life, including meditation and mindfulness.

Made in the USA
Columbia, SC
05 November 2022